BRAIN DISORDERS IN THE ELDERLY: A SELECTED BIBLIOGRAPHY

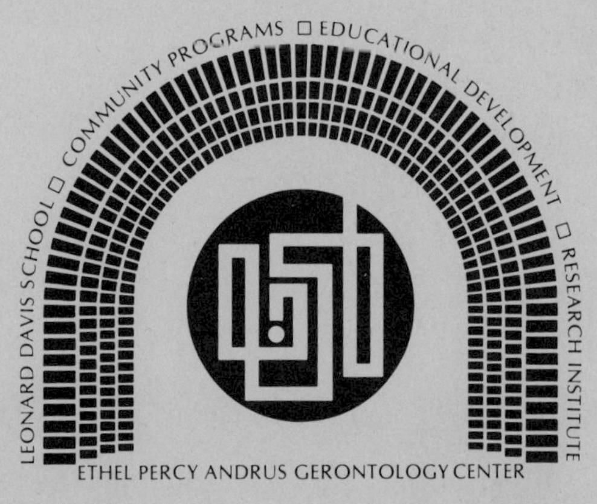

TECHNICAL BIBLIOGRAPHIES

ON AGING

BRAIN DISORDERS IN THE ELDERLY: A SELECTED BIBLIOGRAPHY

EDITED BY:
STEVEN H. ZARIT, PH.D.
and ANITA M. WOODS, M. A.

ETHEL PERCY ANDRUS GERONTOLOGY CENTER
UNIVERSITY OF SOUTHERN CALIFORNIA
UNIVERSITY PARK
LOS ANGELES, CALIFORNIA 90007

This bibliography was compiled under a grant from the National Institute of Mental Health.

Z
6664
.N5
Z37

Published by:

Office of Publications and Media Projects
Richard H. Davis, Ph.D.
Director

Richard Bohen
Bibliographies Project Director
Jean Rarig
Editorial Assistant

The University of Southern California Press
ISBN 0-88474-089-7
Library of Congress Catalog Card Number 79-63569

FOREWORD

The study of aging has been marked in recent years by an increasing optimism about the capabilities of older persons. Research into normal aging processes has established, for example, that in the absence of illness there is far less cognitive decline in old age than had previously been thought. Furthermore, age differences in intelligence have been found to be due to a significant extent to the higher initial levels of functioning of successive cohorts or generations. But gains in knowledge of what is perhaps the most feared and most debilitating problem of old age, the senile brain diseases, is still limited. The situation of older persons with brain impairment is not much different than it was almost 400 years ago when Shakespeare described the last stage of life as "mere oblivion." The growth of knowledge in this area and its practical applications represent a major challenge to the gerontological sciences.

The senile brain syndromes of old age will be examined at various levels in this bibliography. The first three parts cover basic research. First, there will be a review of general, descriptive articles and books that provide an overview of the symptoms, etiology, and prevalence of senile brain syndromes in the elderly. The second section presents biological studies, including pathological, physiological, biochemical and genetic aspects. In the third section, behavioral research is surveyed, including cognitive and psychophysiological aspects of brain syndrome as well as other behavioral manifestations.

The fourth part of the bibliography deals with acute senile brain syndromes. While often reversible and not leading to diffuse brain damage, the acute brain syndromes are not typically given much attention. Because of the prevailing expectation that all older persons are senile, symptoms of acute senile brain syndromes are often mistaken for signs of senile dementia. It has been estimated that as high as one fourth of all those persons diagnosed as having chronic brain syndrome have some reversible aspect of their illness. Yet despite the potential for treatment of acute brain syndromes, there is not an extensive literature on this topic and relatively few systematic investigations have been made.

In the fifth section there will be consideration of the problems of diagnosis and assessment from both medical and behavioral perspectives. The question in diagnostic studies is often how much cognitive change, or how much atrophy on a CAT scan or on some other measure, is sufficient to indicate a senile brain syndrome. While there is some degree of controversy in the area, the absence of specific and effective treatments for such problems as the Alzheimer's-like process of cerebral atrophy, make the distinctions raised in many diagnostic studies somewhat arbitrary at best. Reliable signs of impairment have been established when there are significant amounts of diffuse brain damage, but the development of procedures that detect the senile brain diseases in their early stages has been confounded both by the fact of varying initial levels of ability of individuals and the differences in adaptations that two persons may show to similar processes and amounts of brain damage.

The sixth section includes studies of rehabilitation and management. The first half looks at the sizable amount of drug research that has been conducted in recent years, which has indicated only limited benefits thus far. Behavioral programs of intervention have for the most part emphasized the management of the institutionalized older person. There are, however, many older persons with severe brain impairments who continue to reside in community settings. It has been estimated that there may be as many as three individuals outside nursing homes with senile brain disease for every institutionalized person, and these community-living elderly have deficits as great as those in nursing homes. There clearly needs to be more attention given in the future to those impaired older persons living in the community.

Certain topics have not been covered in this bibliography. The problems of alcoholism and brain damage have not been included, since this topic is so extensive as to warrant its own bibliography. Similarly, Parkinson's disease and the dementia that sometimes results from it have not been reviewed. However, because of the potential relation of the pre-senile dementias such as Alzheimer's and Pick's diseases to senile dementia, articles on these topics have been incorporated into this bibliography.

The method of this bibliography has been to use computerized searches of medical and scientific literature for the period of 1966–1978. Some earlier articles which were judged by the editors to have had important influence have also been included. Both foreign and English language journals have been surveyed but, because of the difficulties in obtaining many of the foreign publications, only a sampling of articles was included in the final selection.

Searches of the following indexing systems were made: Medline; Excerpta Medica; and Psychological Abstracts.

Key words used in conducting the searches included: organic psychoses; organic brain syndromes; chronic brain disease; symptomatic psychoses; senile psychoses; senile dementia; pre-senile dementia; Alzheimer's Disease; Pick's Disease, toxic psychoses; nonpsychotic organic brain syndrome; confusion; delirium; memory disorders; and cerebral arteriosclerosis.

We especially wish to thank Vic Lamanuzzi for his many hours of assistance and his timely words of encouragement. Our thanks also go to Dr. Judy Aklonis for her editorial assistance and encouragement, and to Dick Baumann for his outstanding technical assistance on this project.

This bibliography was developed in connection with the project to produce the *Handbook of Mental Health and Aging,* which is supported by a contract from the National Institute of Mental Health (278-76-0056 SM). The preparation of this manuscript was supported in part by a contract from the National Institute of Mental Health (PLD0864778).

CONTENTS

I. GENERAL

A. BOOKS

Allison, R. S. *The Senile Brain: A Clinical Study.* Baltimore, Md.: Williams & Wilkins, 1962.

Bender, M. B. *Disorders in Perception.* Springfield, Ill.: Charles C. Thomas, 1952.

Birren, J. E., & Sloane, R. B. (Eds.), *Handbook of Mental Health and Aging.* Englewood Cliffs: Prentice-Hall, (in press).

Busse, E. W., & Pfeiffer, E. *Mental Illness in Later Life.* Washington: American Psychiatric Association, 1973.

Butler, R. N., & Lewis M. I. *Aging and Mental Health: Positive Psychosocial Approaches.* St. Louis: Mosby, 1977.

Eisdorfer, C., & Friedel, R. O. (Eds.). *Cognitive and Emotional Disturbance in the Elderly: Clinical Issues.* Chicago: Year Book Medical Publishers, Inc., 1977.

Freedman, D. K. *Acute Organic Disorder Accompanied by Mental Symptoms.* Sacramento, Calif.: Department of Mental Hygiene, 1965.

Himwich, H. E. *Brain Metabolism and Cerebral Disorders.* New York: Spectrum Publications, 1976. (2nd edition)

Lawton, M. P., & Lawton, F. G. (Eds.). *Mental Impairment in the Aged.* Philadelphia: Philadelphia Geriatric Center, 1965.

Lishman, W. A. *Organic Psychiatry: The Psychological Consequences of Cerebral Disorder.* Oxford: Blackwell Scientific Publications, 1978.

Miller, E. *Abnormal Aging: The Psychology of Senile and Presenile Dementia.* New York: Wiley, 1977.

Muller, C., & Ciompi, L. *Senile Dementia: Clinical and Therapeutic Aspects.* Bern: H. Huber, 1968.

Nandy, K. (Ed.). *Senile Dementia: A Biomedical Approach.* New York: Elsevier/North-Holland Biomedical Press, 1978.

Nandy, K., & Sherwin, I. (Eds.). *The Aging Brain and Senile Dementia.* New York: Plenum Press, 1977.

Ordy, J. M., & Brizzee, K. R. (Eds.). *Neurobiology of Aging: An Interdisciplinary Life-Span Approach.* New York: Plenum Press, 1975.

Pearce, J., & Miller, E. *Clinical Aspects of Dementia.* London: Bailliere and Tindall, 1973.

Post, F. *The Clinical Psychiatry of Late Life.* Oxford: Pergamon Press, 1965.

Reitan, R. M., & Davison, L. A. (Eds.). *Clinical Neuropsychology: Current Status and Applications.* New York: Wiley, 1974.

Slaby, A. E., & Wyatt, R. J. *Dementia in the Presenium.* Springfield, Ill.: Charles C. Thomas, 1974.

Smith, W. L., & Kinsbourne, M. *Aging and Senile Dementia.* New York: Spectrum Publications, 1977.

Storandt, M., Siegler, I. C., & Elias, M. F. (Eds.). *The Clinical Psychology of Aging.* New York: Plenum Press, 1978.

Talland, G. *Deranged Memory: A Psychonomic Study of the Amnesic Syndrome.* New York: Academic Press, 1965.

Terry, R. D., & Gershon, S. (Eds.). *Neurobiology of Aging.* New York: Raven Press, 1976.

Weinstein, E. A., & Kahn, R. L. *Denial of Illness: Symbolic and Physiological Aspects.* Springfield, Ill.: Charles C. Thomas, 1955.

Wells, C. E., (Ed.). *Dementia.* Philadelphia: Davis, 1977.

Whitehead, A. *In the Service of Old Age: The Welfare of Psychogeriatric Patients.* Baltimore: Penguin Books, 1970.

Wolstenholme, G. E. W., & O'Connor, M. *Alzheimer's Disease and Related Conditions: CIBA Foundation Symposium.* London: Churchill, 1970.

B. ARTICLES

Akesson, H. O. Senile and arteriosclerotic psychosis. A population study. *Lakartidningen,* 1969, 66(2), 118–124.

Alexander, D. A. "Senile dementia": A changing perspective. *British Journal of Psychiatry,* 1972, 121(561), 207–214.

Aring, C. D. On aging, senescence, and senility. *Annals of Internal Medicine,* 1972, 77, 137–140.

Armstrong, P. W. Comment: More thoughts on senility. *Gerontologist,* 1978, 18(3), 315–316.

Barrett, R. E. Dementia in adults. *Med. Clin. North. Am.,* 1972, 56(6), 1405–1418.

Barton, R. Organic mental disorder (organic brain syndrome). *Practitioner,* 1976, 217(1297), 91–99.

Beighton, P. H., & Lindenberg, R. Alzheimer's disease in multiple members of a family. *Birth Defects,* 1971, 7, 232–233.

Benson, D. F. Normal pressure hydrocephalus: A controversial entity. *Geriatrics,* 1974, 29, 125–132.

Bergmann, K. The epidemiology of senile dementia. *British Journal of Psychiatry,* 1975, 9, 100–109.

Bergmann, K. The epidemiology of senile dementia. *British Journal of Hospital Medicine,* 1969, 2, 727–732.

Bousser, M. G. Modern concepts of "cerebrovascular dementia." *Encephale,* 1977, *3*(4), 357–372.

Brahm, J., Front, D., Sarova-Pinhas, I., Kosary, I. Z., & Czerniak, P. Brain atrophy, hydrocephalus and dementia in adults. *Israel Journal of Medical Sciences,* 1969, *5*(6), 1213–1218.

Brand, F. N., & Gorwitz, K. Relationship of cerebrovascular disease to senile, presenile and cerebral arteriosclerotic dementia. *Journal of Chronic Diseases,* 1971, *24*(9), 569–583.

Brink, T. L. The battle against senility. *Mental Health,* 1977, *61*(2), 11. (Summer-Fall)

Brody, E. M., Kleban, M., Woldow, A., & Freeman, L. Survival and death in the mentally impaired aged. *Journal of Chronic Diseases,* 1975, *28*(7–8), 389–399.

Bucci, L. Senile psychosis and paraphrenia: Some theoretical and practical considerations. *International Journal of Neuropsychiatry,* 1966, *1*(6), 561–566.

Busse, E. W. Mental disorders in later life: Organic brain syndrome. In E. W. Busse & E. Pfeiffer (Eds.), *Mental Illness in Later Life.* Washington, D.C.: American Psychiatric Association, 1973.

Cardiogenic dementia (editorial). *Lancet,* 1977, *1*(8001), 27–28.

Charlton, M. H. Presenile dementia. *New York State Journal of Medicine,* 1975, *75*(9), 1493–1495.

Craigie, H., Robinson, R. A., Henderson, J. H., Williamson, J., Anderson, W. F., & Timbury, G. C. The confused elderly. *Health Bulletin,* 1969, *27*(2), 9–16.

Cramond, W. A. Organic psychosis. *British Medical Journal,* 1968, *4*(629), 497–500.

Cubitt, T., & Bowman, M. Uncovering physical illness in elderly patients with dementia (letter). *British Medical Journal,* 1978, *1*(6109), 365.

A curable form of dementia. *Canadian Medical Association Journal,* 1967, *97*(22), 1358–1359.

Davidson, R. The problem of senile dementia. *Nursing Times,* 1978, *74*(22), 932–933.

Dayan, A. D. Editorial: The brain, aging, and dementia. *Psychological Medicine,* 1974, *4*(4), 349–352.

de Fine, O. B. Theoretical and clinical problems of dementia (editorial). *Ugeskrift for Laeger,* 1976, *138*(45), 2819–2820.

Deibel, A. W. Brief notes on brain syndrome in aging persons. *Journal of Psychiatric Nursing,* 1976, *14*(8), 51–52.

Dementia: The quiet epidemic (editorial). *British Medical Journal,* 1978, *1*(6104), 1–2.

Drachman, D. A. The senile patient. *General Practice,* 1967, *36*(4), 78–87.

Dunea, G., Mahurkar, S. D., Mamdani, B., & Smith, E. C. Role of aluminum in dialysis dementia. *Annals of Internal Medicine,* 1978, *88*(4), 502–504.

Editorial: Organic psychosis. *British Medical Journal,* 1974, *3*(925), 214–215.

Feldshuh, B., Sillen, J., Parker, B., & Frosch, W. The nonpsychotic organic brain syndrome. *American Journal of Psychiatry,* 1973, *130*(9), 1026–1029.

Fisch, M., Goldfarb, A. I., & Shahinian, S. P. Chronic brain syndrome in the community aged. *Archives of General Psychiatry,* 1968, *18,* 739–745.

Gooddy, W. Introduction to the problems of dementia. *Proceedings of the Australian Association of Neurology,* 1969, *6,* 9–11.

Gosch, H. H. Normal pressure hydrocephalus. A treatable cause of dementia. *Journal of the Florida Medical Association,* 1976, *63*(11), 863–864.

Granacher, R. P. The Capgras syndrome in old age (letter). *American Journal of Psychiatry,* 1978, *135*(6), 758–759.

Gruenberg, D. Epidemiology of senile dementia. In R. Katzman & R. Terry (Eds.), *Alzheimer's disease, Senile Dementia, and Related Disorders.* New York: Raven Press, in press.

Gruenberg, E. M. On the frequency of geriatric psychoses by age and sex. *Interdisciplinary Topics in Gerontology,* 1969, *3,* 45–49.

Gustafson, L., & Hagberg, B. Dementia with onset in the presenile period. A cross-sectional study. *Acta Psychiatrica Scandinavica,* 1975, *257,* 3–71. (Supplement)

Hachinski, V. C., Lassen, N. A., & Marshall, J. Multi-infarct dementia. A cause of mental deterioration in the elderly. *Lancet,* 1974, *2,* 207–210.

Hader, M. Organic brain disease and depressive reactions of later life. *Canadian Psychiatric Association,* 1966, *11,* 317–323. (Page Supplement)

Harlan, B. Senile dementia: An increasing problem. *South Dakota Journal of Medicine,* 1976, *29*(6), 5–8.

Hellebrant, F. A. Comment: The senile dement in our midst. A look at the other side of the coin. *Gerontologist,* 1978, *18,* 67–70.

Hill, M. E., Lougheed, W. M., & Barnett, H. J. A treatable form of dementia due to normal pressure, communicating hydrocephalus. *Canadian Medical Association Journal,* 1967, *97*(22), 1309–1320.

Hughes, W. Alzheimer's disease. *Gerontologia Clinica*(Basel), 1970, *12*(3), 129–148.

Isaacs, B., & Caird, F. I. Brain failure: A contribution to the terminology of mental abnormality in old age. *Age and Ageing,* 1976, *5*(4), 241–244.

Jacobson, S. B. Geriatric psychiatry today. *Bulletin of the New York Academy of Medicine,* 1978, *54*(6), 568–572.

Kahn, R. L. Psychological aspects of aging. In I. Rossman (Ed.), *Clinical Geriatrics.* Philadelphia: J. B. Lippincott, 1971.

Kaszniak, A. W., Fox, J., Gandell, D. L., Garron, D. C., Huckman, M. S., & Ramsey, R. G. Predictors of mortality in presenile and senile dementia. *Annals of Neurology,* 1978, *3*(3), 246–252.

Katzman, R. Editorial: The prevalence and malignancy of Alzheimer disease: A major killer. *Archives of Neurology,* 1976, *33*(4), 217–218.

Kay, D. W. Senility. *Community Health*(Bristol), 1970, *2*(3), 127–132.

Kay, D. W. K. Epidemiological aspects of organic brain disease in the aged. *Advances in Behavioral Biology,* 1972, *3,* 15–27.

Kay, D. W. K. Outcome and cause of death in mental disorders of old age: A long-term follow-up of functional and organic psychoses. *Acta Psychiatrica Scandinavica,* 1962, *38,* 249–276.

Kay, D. W. K., Beamish, P., & Roth, M. Old age mental disorders in New Castle upon Tyne, Part I: A study of prevalence. *British Journal of Psychiatry,* 1964, *110,* 146–158.

Kay, D. W. K., Beamish, P., & Roth, M. R. Old age mental disorders in Newcastle-upon-Tyne, Part II. A study of possible social and medical causes. *British Journal of Psychiatry,* 1964, *110,* 668–682.

Kay, D. W. K., Roth, M., & Hopkins, B. Affective disorders in the senium: I. Their association with organic cerebral degeneration. *Journal of Mental Science,* 1955, *101,* 302–318.

Kent, S. Classifying and treating organic brain syndromes. *Geriatrics,* 1977, *32*(9), 87–89.

Korkushko, O. V. Premature aging and its prevention. *Feldsher i Akusherka*(Rus.), 1978, *43*(4), 40–44.

Kral, V. A. Psychiatric problems in the aged: A reconsideration. *Canadian Medical Association Journal,* 1973, *108*(5), 584. (Passim.)

Kral, V. A. Senile dementia and normal aging. *Canadian Psychiatric Association Journal,* 1972, *17*(2), (Supplement 2:ss25-).

Larsson, T. Aetiology and epidemiology of senile dementia. In P. From Hansen (Ed.), *Age with a Future.* Copenhagen: Munksgaard, 1964.

Larsson, T., Sjogren, T., & Jacobsen, G. Senile dementia: A clinical sociomedical and genetic study. *Acta Psychiatrica Scandinavica,* 1963, *39,* 1–259. (Supplement 167)

Lauter, H. Late forms of Alzheimer's disease and their relationship to senile dementia. *Psychiatria Clinica*(Basel), 1970, *3*(3), 169–189.

Lijtmaer, H., Fuld, P. A., & Katzman, R. Letter: Prevalence and malignancy of Alzheimer disease. *Archives of Neurology,* 1976, *33*(4), 304.

Lissitz, S. The challenge of the senile aged. *Gerontologist,* 1969, *9*(2), 114–119.

Lowe, B. D. Senile? *Imprint,* 1978, *25,* 46;71.

Lying-Tunell, U., Bergquist, D., Bohmer, G., Malmlund, H. O., Marions, O., & Soderborg, B. Studies in presenile dementia. *Acta Neurologica Scandinavica,* 1970, *46,* (Supplement 43:90–92).

Macmillan, D. Features of senile breakdown. *Geriatrics,* 1969, *24*(3), 109–118.

The many faces of dementia. *Canadian Medical Association Journal,* 1971, *105*(11), 1127.

Marsden, C. D., & Harrison, M. J. G. Presenile dementia. *British Medical Journal,* 1972, *3,* 50–55.

Marttila, R. J. & Rinne, U. K. Dementia in Parkinson's disease. *Acta Neurologica Scandinavica,* 1976, *54*(5), 431–441.

McDermott, J. R., Smith, A. I., Iqbal, K., & Wisniewski, H. M. Aluminium and Alzheimer's disease (letter). *Lancet,* 1977, *2*(8040), 710–711.

McKechnie, A. A., Foster, E. M., Bergmann, K., & Kay, D. W. Psychiatric illness in the elderly. A comparison of GP records and survey findings. *Gerontology,* 1978, *24*(4), 293–298.

Meyer, J. S. Summary of the Seventh International Salzburg Conference on Cerebral Vascular Disease, September 25–29, 1974. *Stroke,* 1975, *6*(2), 109–115.

Miller, E. Dementia as an accelerated ageing of the nervous system: Some psychological and methodological considerations. *Age and Ageing,* 1974, *3*(4), 197–202.

Muller, C. The problem of the interference of senile deterioration with preexisting psychoses. *Encephale,* 1970, *59,* 81–89.

Muller, H., Grad, B., & Engelsmann, F. Biological and psychological predictors of survival in a psychogeriatric population. *Journal of Gerontology,* 1975, *30,* 47–52.

Neuman, M. A., & Cohn, R. Prevalence and malignancy of Alzheimer disease (letter). *Archives of Neurology,* 1976, *33*(10), 730.

Payne, R., Gibson, F. E., & Pittard, B. B. Social influences in senile psychosis. *Sociological Symposium,* 1969, *2,* 137–146.

Pearce, J. The extrapyramidal disorder of Alzheimer's disease. *European Neurology,* 1974, *12*(2), 94–103.

Peck, A., Wolloch, L., & Rodstein, M. Mortality of the aged with chronic brain syndrome. *Journal of the American Geriatrics Society,* 1973, *21,* 264–270.

Peck, A. Wolloch, L., & Rodstein, M. Mortality of the aged with chronic brain syndrome: Further observations in a five-year study. *Journal of the American Geriatrics Society,* 1978, *26*(4), 170–176.

Perez, R., Wamba, M., & Gomez, G. Psychotic and nonpsychotic organic brain syndromes in the psychiatric service of a general hospital. *Archivos de Neurobiologia,* 1977, *40*(2), 53–78.

Perlo, V. P. Hydrocephalus with dementia. *New England Journal of Medicine,* 1970, *283*(12), 654–655.

Pinel, C. Pick's disease. *Nursing Times,* 1977, *73*(43), 1675–1676.

Poser, C. M. The presenile dementias. *Journal of the American Medical Association,* 1975, *233*, 81–84.

Post, F. Dementia, depression and pseudodementia. In D. F. Benson & D. Blumer (Eds.), *Psychiatric Aspects of Neurologic Disease.* New York: Grune & Stratton, 1975.

Post, F. The development and progress of senile dementia in relationship to the functional psychiatric disorders of later life. In C. Muller & L. Ciompi (Eds.), *Senile Dementia.* Bern: Hans Huber, 1968.

Reichel, W. Organic brain syndromes in the aged. *Hospital Practice,* 1976, *11*(5), 119–125.

Reid, A. H., & Aungle, P. G. Dementia in ageing mental defectives: A clinical psychiatric study. *Journal of Mental Deficiency Research,* 1974, *18*, 15–23.

Reimann, H., & Hafner, H. Mental disorders of the elderly in Mannheim: An investigation of incidence rate. *Social Psychiatry,* 1972, *7*, 53–69.

Rivera, V. W., & Meyer, J. S. Dementia and cerebrovascular disease. In J. S. Meyer (Ed.), *Modern Concepts of Cerebrovascular Disease.* New York: Spectrum, 1975.

Rogers, W. G., & Miller, W. C. Alzheimer's disease: A review of recent studies. *Journal of the South Carolina Medical Association,* 1972, *68*(10), 383–386.

Roth, M. The natural history of mental disorder in old age. *Journal of Mental Science,* 1955, *101*, 281–301.

Rubens, R. D. Reversible organic dementia due to normal-pressure communicating hydrocephalus. *Proceedings of the Royal Society of Medicine,* 1970, *63*(12), 1308–1309.

Salmon, J. H. Senile and presenile dementia. *Geriatrics,* 1969, *24*, 67–72.

Schaumburg, H. H., & Suzuki, K. Nonspecific familial presenile dementia. *Journal of Neurology, Neurosurgery, and Psychiatry,* 1968, *31,* 479–486.

Shulman, R. The present status of vitamin B 12 and folic acid deficiency in psychiatric illness. *Canadian Psychiatric Association Journal,* 1972, *17*(3), 205–216.

Sloane, R. B. Organic Brain Syndrome. In J. E. Birren & R. B. Sloane (Eds.), *Handbook of Mental Health and Aging.* Englewood Cliffs: Prentice-Hall, in press.

Smith, A. Ambiguities in concepts and studies of brain damage and organicity. *The Journal of Nervous and Mental Disease,* 1962, *135,* 311–326.

Sourander, P., & Walinder, J. Hereditary multi-infarct dementia. Morphological and clinical studies of a new disease. *Acta Neuropathologica,* 1977, *39*(3), 247–254.

Stevens, D. L., Hewlett, R. H. & Brownell, B. Chronic familial vascular encephalopathy (letter). *Lancet,* 1977, *1*(8026), 1364–1365.

Stochdorph, O. Gerontopsychiatric syndrome in virus diseases of the brain. In W. Doberauer, (Ed.), *Scriptum Geriatricum.* Munchen: Urban & Schwarzenberg, 1975.

Storey, P. Organic psychoses. *Practitioner,* 1973, *210*(255), 79–85.

Sugimura, H. Clinical psychology of dementia: Psychological approach in the study of senile dementia. *Japanese Journal of the Nursing Art,* 1976, *22*(7), 25–31.

Szanto, S. Dementia in the elderly. *Nursing Mirror,* 1975, *140* (23), 64–65.

Terry, R. D. Dementia. A brief and selective view. *Archives of Neurology,* 1976, *33,* 1–4.

Tissot, R. On the nosological identity of senile dementia and of Alzheimer's disease. In C. Muller & L. Ciompi (Eds.), *Senile Dementia.* Bern-Stuttgart: Hans Huber, 1968.

Tolwinski, T., & Strugulewska, G. Clinical follow-up of senile psychosis treated at the Choroszcz hospital from 1960 to 1970. *Psychiatria Polska,* 1973, *7,* 29–37.

Tomlinson, B. E. The pathology of dementia. *Contemporary Neurological Series,* 1977, *15,* 113–153.

Unterberger, H., & Reynolds, A. S. A study of chronic organic brain disorders in a psychiatric hospital. *Behavioral Neuropsychiatry,* 1969, *1*(2), 18–22.

Vijayan, N., Cuanang, J. R., & Dreyfus, P. M. Dementia. Current concepts. *California Medicine,* 1969, *111*(3), 208–216.

Waldton, S. Clinical observations of impaired cranial nerve function in senile dementia. *Acta Psychiatrica Scandinavica,* 1974, *50*(5), 539–547.

Walsh, A. C. Senile dementia. *Journal of the South Carolina Medical Association,* 1968, 64(3), 85–93.

Wang, H. S. Dementia in old age. *Contemporary Neurology Series,* 1977, *15,* 15–27.

Wang, H. S. Organic brain syndrome in the elderly. A reevaluation of concepts. *Postgraduate Medicine,* 1972, *51*(2), 237–241.

Wang, H. S. Organic brain syndromes. In E. W. Busse & E. Pfeiffer (Eds.), *Behavior and Adaptation in Late Life.* Boston: Little & Brown, 1969.

Wang, H. S., & Busse, E. W. Dementia in old age. *Contemporary Neurology Series,* 1971, *9,* 151–162.

Wells, C. E. Dementia reconsidered. *Archives of General Psychiatry,* 1972, *26*(4), 385–388.

Wells, C. E. Dementia: Definition and description. *Contemporary Neurology Series,* 1977, *15,* 1–14.

Wells, C. E. Role of stroke in dementia. *Stroke,* 1978, *9,* 1–3.

Wertheimer, J., & Brull, J. Methodology of a long-term study of senile dementia. *Schweizer Arch. fuer Neurologie Neurochirurgie und Psychiatrie,* 1977, *120*(2), 309–322.

When is dementia presenile? *British Medical Journal,* 1972, *2* (811), 465.

Whitehead, A. The prediction of outcome in elderly psychiatric patients. *Psychological Medicine,* 1976, *6*(3), 469–479.

Wilkins, R. H., & Brody, I. A. Alzheimer's disease. *Archives of Neurology,* 1969, *21,* 109–110.

Wood, R. A. Psychological medicine: Organic illness. *British Medical Journal,* 1975, *1*(5960), 723–726.

II. BIOLOGICAL STUDIES

A. NEUROANATOMY

Ball, M. J. Neurofibrillary tangles in the dementia of normal pressure hydrocephalus. *Canadian Journal of Neurological Sciences,* 1976, *3*(4), 227–235.

Ball, M. J. Neuronal loss, neurofibrillary tangles and granulo-vacuolar degeneration in the hippocampus with ageing and dementia. A quantitative study. *Acta Neuropathologica*(Berlin), 1977, *37*(2), 111–118.

Ball, M. J. Topographic distribution of neurofibrillary tangles and granulovacuolar degeneration in hippocampal cortex of aging and demented patients. A quantitative study. *Acta Neuropathologica,* 1978, *42*(2), 73–80.

Ball, M. J., & Lo, P. Granulovacuolar degeneration in the ageing brain and in dementia. *Journal of Neuropathology and Experimental Neurology,* 1977, *36*(3), 474–487.

Beskow, J., Hassler, O., & Ottosson, J. O. Cerebral arterial deformities in relation to senile deterioration. *Acta Psychiatrica Scandinavica,* 1971, *221,* 111–. (Supplement)

Bianchi, C., Brollo, A., & D'Osualdo, E. Amyloid senile plaques in late senility. *Pathologica*(Ita), 1977, *68*(993), 369–372.

Bignami, A. Our present knowledge of the pathology of dementias. *Modern Trends in Neurology,* 1975, *6, 1*–16.

Brun, A., & Gustafson, L. Distribution of cerebral degeneration in Alzheimer's disease. A clinico-pathological study. *Archiv fuer Psychiatrie und Nervenkrankheiten,* 1976, *223,* 15–33.

Burger, P. C., & Vogel, F. S. The development of the pathologic changes of Alzheimer's disease and senile dementia in patients with Down's syndrome. *American Journal of Pathology,* 1973, *73*(2), 457–476.

Colon, E. J. The cerebral cortex in presenile dementia. A quantitative analysis. *Acta Neuropathologica,* 1973, *23*(4), 281–290.

Constantinidis, J., Richard, J., & Tissot, R. Pick's disease: Histological and clinical correlations. *Journal of Neurology, Neurosurgery and Psychiatry,* 1974, *37*(7), 841–847.

Corsellis, J. A. Mental illness and the aging brain: The distribution of pathological change in a mental hospital population. *Maudsley Monographs,* No. 9, 1962.

Corsellis, J. A. The pathology of dementia. *British Journal of Psychiatry,* 1975, *9,* 110–118.

Corsellis, J. A. The pathology of dementia. *British Journal of Hospital Medicine,* 1969, *2,* 695–703.

Davies, P., & Maloney, A. J. Selective loss of central cholinergic neurons in Alzheimer's disease (letter). *Lancet,* 1976, *2* (8000), 1403.

Dayan, A. D. Presenile dementia: Some pathological problems and possibilities. *Proceedings of the Royal Society of Medicine,* 1971, *64*(8), 829–831.

Dayan, A. D. Quantitative histological studies on the aged human brain. II. Senile plaques and neurofibrillary tangles in senile dementia (appendix on their occurrence in Carcinoma). *Acta Neuropathologica,* 1970, *16*(2), 95–102.

Ellis, W. G., McCulloch, J. R., & Corley, C. L. Presenile dementia in Down's syndrome. Ultrastructural identity with Alzheimer's disease. *Neurology,* 1974, *24*(2), 101–106.

Engeset, A. Radiological considerations on the aetiological and anatomical background of presenile dementias. *Acta Neurologica Scandinavica,* 1970, *46,* (Supplement 43:32+).

Field, E. J. Amyloidosis, Alzheimer's disease, and ageing. *Lancet,* 1970, *2,* 780–781.

Gunner-Svensson, F., Andersson, P. G., Jensen, K., & Lorentzen, K. A. Presenile dementia (Alzheimer's and Pick's diseases). A retrospective clinical and patholgoical study. *Acta Neurologica Scandinavica,* 1970, *46,* (Supplement 43:77).

Hanley, T. 'Neuronal fall-out' in the ageing brain: A critical review of the quantitative data. *Age and Ageing,* 1974, *3*(3), 133–151.

Hassler, O. Arterial deformities in senile brains: The occurrence of the deformities in a large autopsy series and some aspects of their functional significance. *Acta Neuropathologica,* 1967, *8*(3), 219–225.

Hassler, O. Vascular changes in senile brains. A micro-angiographic study. *Acta Neuropathologica,* 1965, *5*(1), 40–53.

Hopper, M. W., & Vogel, F. S. The Limbic system in Alzheimer's disease. A neuropathologic investigation. *American Journal of Pathology,* 1976, *85,* 1–20.

Iqbal, K., Wisniewski, H. M., Grundke-Iqbal, I., Korthals, J. K., & Terry, R. D. Chemical pathology of neurofibrils. Neurofibrillary tangles in Alzheimer's presenile-senile dementia. *Journal of Histochemistry and Cytochemistry,* 1975, *23*(7), 563–569.

Ishino, H., & Otsuki, S. Distribution of Alzheimer's neurofibrillary tangles in the basal ganglia and brain stem of progressive supranuclear palsy and Alzheimer's disease. *Folia Psychiatrica et Neurologica Japonica,* 1975, *29*(2), 179–187.

Ishino, H., & Otsuki, S. Frequency of Alzheimer's neurofibrillary tangles in the basal ganglia and brain-stem in Alzheimer's disease, senile dementia and the aged. *Folia Psychiatrica et Neurologica Japonica,* 1975, *29*(3), 279–287.

Jamada, M., & Mehraein, P. Distribution of senile changes in the brain. The part of the limbic system in Alzheimer's disease and senile dementia. *Archiv fuer Psychiatrie und Nerverkrankheiten,* 1968, *211*(3), 308–324.

Jellinger, K. Cerebrovascular amyloidosis with cerebral hemorrhage. *Journal of Neurology,* 1977, *214*(3), 195–206.

Jellinger, K. Neuropathological aspects of dementias resulting from abnormal blood and cerebrospinal fluid dynamics. *Acta Neurological Belgica,* 1976, *76*(2), 83–102.

Kalter, S., & Kelly, S. Alzheimer's disease. Evaluation of immunologic indices. *New York State Journal of Medicine,* 1975, *75*(8), 1222–1225.

Livesley, B. The pathogenesis of brain failure in the aged. *Age and Ageing,* 1977, 9–19. (Supplement)

Mandybur, T. J. The incidence of cerebral amyloid angiopathy in Alzheimer's disease. *Neurology,* 1975 *25*(2), 120–126.

Mehraein, P., Yamada, M., & Tarnowska-Dziduszko, E. Quantitative study on dendrites and dendritic spines in Alzheimer's disease and senile dementia. *Advances in Neurology,* 1975, *12,* 453–458.

Miyakawa, T., Sumiyoshi, S., Murayama, E., & Deshimaru, M. Ultrastructure of capillary plaque-like degeneration in senile dementia. Mechanism of amyloid production. *Acta Neuropathologica*(Berlin), 1974, *29*(3), 229–236.

Morimatsu, M. Pathogenesis of dementia in the aged: Analysis based on the involutional changes and the vascular lesions of the brain. *Japanese Journal of Gerontology,* 1975, *12,* 41–50.

Morimatsu, M., Hirai, S., Muramatsu, A., & Yoshikawa, M. Senile degenerative brain lesions and dementia. *Journal of the American Geriatrics Society,* 1975, *23*(9), 390–406.

Nikaido, T., Austin, J., Trueb, L., Hutchison, J., Rinehart, R., Stuckenbrok, H., & Miles, B. Isolation and preliminary characterization of Alzheimer plaques from presenile and senile dementia. *Trans-American Neurological Association,* 1970, *95,* 47–50.

Sabuncu, N. Quantitative histology of senile psychoses. *Verhandlungen der Deutschen Gesellschaft fuer Pathologie,* 1968, *52,* 250–255.

Scheibel, A. B., & Tomiyasu, U. Dendritic sprouting in Alzheimer's presenile dementia. *Experimental Neurology,* 1978, *60,* 1–8.

Schwartz, P. Pathoanatomic alterations in the aged. *Psychosomatics,* 1967, *8*(4), 12–20. (Page Supplement)

Shefer, V. F. Absolute number of neurons and thickness of the cerebral cortex during aging, senile and vascular dementia, and Pick's and Alzheimer's diseases. *Neuroscience and Behavioral Physiology,* 1973, 6(4), 319–324.

Shefer, V. F. Distribution pattern of nerve cells in cerebral structures in youth, old age, and dementia (senile vascular dementia, Pick's and Alzheimer's diseases). *Arkhiv Anatomii Gistologii i Embriologii,* 1971, 60(6), 94–100.

Shefer, V. F. Hippocampal pathology as one of the possible factors in the pathogenesis of several dementias of old age. *Zhurnal Nevropatologii i Psikhiatrii,* 1976, *76*(7), 1032–1036.

Shibayama, H., & Kitoh, J. Electron microscopic structure of the Alzheimer's neurofibrilalary changes in case of atypical senile dementia. *Acta Neuropathologica,* 1978, *41*(3), 229–234.

Sjogren, H. Presenile-senile brain atrophic syndromes related to micro- and macroscopical analysis and to weight of the brain. A study of 400 cases. *Acta Psychiatrica Scandinavica,* 1965, *41*(3), 446–461.

Sjogren, T., Sjogren, H., & Lindgren, A. G. H. Morbus Alzheimer and morbus Pick. *Acta Psychiatrica et Neurolgica Scandinavica,* 1952, *82,* (Suppl. 82).

Smith, W. T. The pathology of the organic dementias. *Modern Trends in Neurology,* 1970, *5,* 96–126.

Tellez-Nagel, I. Ultrastructure and histochemistry of the dementias. *Psychiatric Forum,* 1973, *4,* 27–38.

Terry, R. D., & Wisniewski, H. M. Pathology and pathogenesis of dementia. In W. S. Fields, (Ed.), *Neurological and Sensory Disorders in the Elderly,* New York: Stratton, 1975.

Tomlinson, B. E., Blessed, G., & Roth, M. Observations on the brains of demented old people. *Journal of Neurological Science,* 1970, *11*(3), 205–242.

Torvik, A. Aspects of the pathology of presenile dementia. *Acta Neurologica Scandinavica,* 1970, *46,* (Supplement 43:19 +).

Wisniewski, H. M., Coblentz, J. M., & Terry, R. D. Pick's disease: A clinical and ultrastructural study. *Archives of Neurology,* 1972, *26*(2), 97–108.

B. NEUROPHYSIOLOGY AND BIOCHEMICAL ASPECTS

Averbukh, E. S., & Shatalova, A. A. Blood and urine catecholamine and histamine concentrations in senile psychoses, *Zhurnal Nevropatologii i Psikhiatrii,* 1970, *70*(6), 888–891.

Banta, R. G., & Markesbery, W. R. Elevated manganese levels associated with dementia and extrapyramidal signs. *Neurology,* 1977, *27*(3), 213–216.

Bock, E., Kristensen, V., & Rafaelsen, O. J. Proteins in serum and cerebrospinal fluid in demented patients. *Acta Neurologica Scandinavica,* 1974, *50,* 91–102.

Bowen, D. M. Biochemistry of dementias. *Proceedings of the Royal Society of Medicine,* 1977, *70*(5), 351–353.

Bowen, D. M., Smith, C. B., & Davison, A. N. Molecular changes in senile dementia. *Brain,* 1973, *96*(4), 849–856.

Bowen, D. M., Smith, C. B., White, P., & Davison, A. N. Neurotransmitter-related enzymes and indices of hypoxia in senile dementia and other abiotrophies. *Brain,* 1976, *99*(3), 459–496.

Bowen, D., White, P., Flack, R., Smith, C., & Davison, A. Brain-decarboxylase activities as indices of pathological change in senile dementia. *Lancet,* 1974, *1*(869), 1247–1249.

Butler, R. N., Dastur, D. K., & Perlin, S. Relationships of senile manifestations and chronic brain syndromes to cerebral circulation and metabolism. *Journal of Psychiatric Research,* 1965, *3*(4), 229–238.

Cherayil, G. D. Fatty acid composition of brain glycolipids in Alzheimer's disease, senile dementia, and cerebrocortical atrophy. *Journal of Lipid Research,* 1968, *9*(2), 207–214.

Cholinergic involvement in senile dementia (editorial). *Lancet,* 1977, *1*(8008), 408.

Constantinidis, J., Richard, J., & Tissot, R. Pick's disease histological and clinical correlations. *European Neurology,* 1974, *11*(4), 208–217.

Cox, J. R., & Orme, J. E. Body water, electrolytes, and psychological test performance in elderly patients. *Gerontologia Clinica,* 1973, *15*(4), 203–208.

Crapper, D. R., Krishnan, S. S., & Dalton, A. J. Brain aluminum distribution in Alzheimer's disease and experimental neurofibrillary degeneration. *Transactions of the American Neurological Association,* 1973, *98,* 17–20.

Crapper, D. R., Krishnan, S. S., & Dalton, A. J. Brain aluminum distribution in Alzheimer's disease and experimental neurofibrillary degeneration. *Science,* 1973, *180*(85), 511–513.

Crapper, D. R., Krishnan, S. S., & Quittkat, S. Aluminum, neurofibrillary degeneration and Alzheimer's disease. *Brain,* 1976, *99*(1), 67–80.

Davies, P. & Verth, A. H. Regional distribution of muscarinic acetylcholine receptor in normal and Alzheimer's-type dementia brains. *Brain Research,* 1977, *138*(2), 385–392.

Dayan, A. D., & Ball, M. J. Histometric observations on the metabolism of tangle-bearing neurons. *Journal of Neurological Sciences,* 1973, *19*(4), 433–436.

Dekoninck, W. J., Collard, M., & Noel, G. Cerebral vasocreactivity in senile dementia. *Gerontology,* 1977, *23*(2), 148–160.

den Velde, W., & Stam, F. C. Some cerebral proteins and enzyme systems in Alzheimer's presenile and senile dementia. *Journal of the American Geriatrics Society,* 1976, *24*(1), 12–16.

Dialysis dementia: Aluminium again (editorial). *Lancet,* 1976, *1*(7955), 349.

Domino, E. F., Krause, R. R., & Bowers, J. Various enzymes involved with putative neurotransmitters. Regional distribution in brain of deceased mentally normal, chronic schizophrenics or organic brain syndrome patients. *Archives of General Psychiatry,* 1973, *29*(2), 195–201.

Duckett, S. Aluminum and Alzheimer disease (letter). *Archives of Neurology,* 1976, *33*(10), 730–731.

Editorial: Cerebral blood flow in dementia. *British Medical Journal,* 1976, *1*(6024), 1487–1488.

Gottfries, C. G., Gottfries, I., & Roos, B. E. Homovanillic acid and 5-hydroxyindoleacetic acid in the cerebrospinal fluid of patients with senile dementia, presenile dementia and parkinsonism. *Journal of Neurochemistry,* 1969, *16*(9), 1341–1345.

Harris, R. The relationship between organic brain disease and physical status. In C. M. Gaitz (Ed.), *Aging and the Brain,* New York: Plenum Press, 1972.

Hattangadi, S. B., Grad, B., Beckett, M. E., & Csank, J. Z. Some clinical and biochemical variables in patients with chronic brain syndrome. *Journal of the American Geriatrics Society,* 1973, *21*(10), 460–464.

Iqbal, K., Wisniewski, H. M., Shelanski, M. L., Brostoff, S., Liwnicz, B. H., & Terry, R. D. Protein changes in senile dementia. *Brain Research,* 1974, *77*(2), 337–343.

Kalter, S., & Kelly, S. Alzheimer's disease. Evaluation of immunologic indices. *New York State Journal of Medicine,* 1975, *75*(8), 1222–1225.

Lambert, P. A., & Bouchardy, M. Can psychiatric disorders of the aged be influenced by affecting the cerebral circulation? *Semaine Therapie*(Fr.), 1968, *44*(10), 654–655.

Levy, R. The neurophysiology of dementia. *British Journal of Psychiatry,* 1975, *9,* 119–123.

Levy, R., Isaacs, A., & Hawks, G. Neurophysiological correlates of senile dementia. I. Motor and sensor nerve conduction velocity. *Psychological Medicine,* 1970, *1,* 40–47.

Libikova, H., Pogady, J., Wiedermann, V., & Breier, S. Search for herpetic antibodies in the cerebrospinal fluid of senile dementia and mental retardation. *Acta Virologica,* 1975, *19*(6), 493–495.

Mayer, P. P., Chughtai, M. A., & Cape, R. D. An immunological approach to dementia in the elderly. *Age and Ageing,* 1976, *5*(3), 164–170.

McNamara, J. O., & Appel, S. H. Biochemical approaches to dementia. *Contemporary Neurology Series,* 1977, *15,* 155–168.

Miner, G. D., Trapp, G. A., McSwigan, J., & Heston, L. L. Alzheimer's disease: Human brain protein 13–7. *Journal of Neurochemistry,* 1976, *26*(3), 605–607.

Miyakawa, T., Sumiyoshi, S., Murayama, E., & Deshimaru, M. Ultrastructure of capillary plaque-like degeneration in senile dementia. Mechanism of amyloid production. *Acta Neuropathologica,* 1974, *29*(3), 229–236.

Nikaido, T., Austin, J., Trueb, L., & Rinehart, R. Studies in ageing of the brain. II. Microchemical analysis of the nervous system in Alzheimer patients. *Archives of Neurology,* 1972, *27*(6), 549–554.

O'Brien, M. D., & Mallett, B. L. Cerebral cortex perfusion rates in dementia. *Journal of Neurology, Neurosurgery and Psychiatry,* 1970, *33*(4), 497–500.

Oksova, E. E. Nucleic acid concentration in cerebral cortex nerve cells in senile dementia. *Zhurnal Nevropatologii i Psikhiatrii,* 1973, *73*(7), 1038–1040.

Pavlova, S. I. Changes in teh blood clotting system of patients with atherosclerotic and senile dementias. *Zhurnal Nevropatologii i Psikhiatrii,* 1978, *78*(3), 409–412.

Perry, E. K., Perry, R. H., Blessed, G., & Tomlinson, B. E. Necropsy evidence of central cholinergic deficits in senile dementia (letter). *Lancet,* 1977, *1*(8004), 189.

Perry, E., Gibson, P., Blessed, G., Perry, R., & Tomlinson, B. Neurotransmitter enzyme abnormalities in senile dementia. Choline acetyltransferase and glutamic acid decarboxylase activities in necropsy brain tissue. *Journal of Neurological Sciences,* 1977, *34*(2), 247–265.

Roos, D., & Willanger, R. Various degrees of dementia in a selected group of gastrectomized patients with low serum B12. *Acta Neurologica Scandinavica,* 1977, *55*(5), 363–376.

Roos, R. P. & Johnson, R. T. Viruses and dementia. *Contemporary Neurology Series,* 1977, *15*, 93–112.

Shaw, D. M., *et al.* Folate and amine metabolites in senile dementia: A combined trial and biochemical study. *Psychological Medicine,* 1971, *1*(2), 166–171.

Shefer, V. F. Absolute number of neurons and thickness of the cerebral cortex during aging, senile and vascular dementia, and Pick's and Alzheimer's diseases. *Neurosci. Behav. Physiology,* 1973, *6*(4), 319–324.

Szanto, S. Blood platelet behaviour in primary neuronal and vascular dementia. *Age and Ageing,* 1972, *1*(4), 207–212.

Waldton, S. Clinical observations of impaired cranial nerve function in senile dementia. *Acta Psychiatrica Scandinavica,* 1974, *50*(5), 539–547.

White, P., Hiley, C. R., Goodhardt, M. J., Carrasco, L. H., Keet, J. P., Williams, I. E., & Bowen, D. M. Neocortical cholinergic neurons in elderly people. *Lancet,* 1977, *1*(8013), 668–671.

Whittingham, S., Lennon, V., MacKay, I. R., Davies, G. V., & Davies, B. Absence of brain antibodies in senile dementia. *British Journal of Psychiatry,* 1970, *116*(533), 447–448.

C. GENETICS

Akesson, H. O. A population study of senile and arteriosclerotic psychoses. *Human Heredity,* 1969, *19*(5), 546–566.

Brun, A., Gustafson, L., & Mitelman, F. Normal chromosome banding pattern in Alzheimer's disease. *Gerontology,* 1978, *24*(5), 369–372.

Cohen, D. A behavioral-chromosome relationship in the elderly: A critical review of a biobehavioral hypothesis. *Experimental Aging Research,* 1976, *2*(3), 271–287.

Heston, L. L. The clinical genetics of Pick's disease. *Acta Psychiatrica Scandinavica,* 1978, *57*(3), 202–206.

Heston, L. L., & Mastri, A. R. The genetics of Alzheimer's disease: Associations with hematologic malignancy and Down's syndrome. *Archives of General Psychiatry,* 1977, *34*(8), 976–981.

Jarvik, L. F., Altshuler, K. Z., Kato, T., & Blumner, B. Organic brain syndrome and chromosome loss in aged twins. *Diseases of the Nervous System,* 1971, *32*(3), 159–170.

Mark, J., & Brun, A. Chromosomal deviations in Alzheimer's disease compared to those in senescence and senile dementia. *Gerontologia Clinica,* 1973, *15*(5), 253–258.

Nielsen, J. Chromosomes in senile dementia. *British Journal of Psychiatry,* 1968, *114*(508), 303–309.

Nielsen, J. Chromosomes in senile, presenile, and arteriosclerotic dementia. *Journal of Gerontology,* 1970, *25*(4), 312–315.

Opden Velde, W., & Stam, F. C. Haptoglobin types in Alzheimer's disease and senile dementia. *British Journal of Psychiatry,* 1973, *122*(568), 331–336.

Reighton, P. H., & Lindenberg, R. Alzheimer's disease in multiple members of a family. *Birth Defects,* 1971, *7,* 232–233.

III. BEHAVIORAL STUDIES

A. COGNITIVE STUDIES

Aggernaes, A., & Myscheitzky, A. Experienced reality in somatic patients more than 65 years old. A comparative study of disturbed and clear, but demented states of consciousness. *Acta Psychiatrica Scandinavica,* 1976, *54*(4), 225–237.

Alexander, D. A. Attention dysfunction in senile dementia. *Psychological Reports,* 1973, *32*(1), 229–230.

Alexander, D. A. Some tests of intelligence and learning for elderly psychiatric patients: A validation study. *British Journal of Social and Clinical Psychology,* 1973, *12*(2), 188–193.

Barker, M. G., & Lawson, J. S. Nominal aphasia in dementia. *British Journal of Psychiatry,* 1968, *114*(516), 1351–1356.

Ben-Yishay, Y., Diller, L., Mandleberg, I., Gordon, W., & Gerstman, L. Similarities and differences in block design performance between older normal and brain-injured persons: A task analysis. *Journal of Abnormal Psychology,* 1971, *78*, 17–25.

Bender, M. B. The incidence and type of perceptual deficiencies in the aged. In W. S. Fields (Ed.), *Neurological and Sensory Disorders in the Elderly.* New York: Stratton Intercontinental, 1975.

Bettner, L. G., Jarvik, L. F., & Blum, J. E. Stroop color-word test, non-psychotic organic brain syndrome, and chromosome loss in aged twins. *Journal of Gerontology,* 1971, *26*(4), 458–469.

Bleikher, V. M., & Mashek, I. Experience in the use of psychometric studies in memory in cerebral arteriosclerosis. *Zhurnal Nevropatologii i Psikhiatrii,* 1974, *74*(2), 251–255.

Bleikher, V. M., & Mashek, I. Pathopsychological study of memory in cerebral arteriosclerosis. *Zhurnal Nevropatologii i Psykhiatrii,* 1973, *73*(9), 1358–1363.

Bolton, N., Britton, P. G., & Savage, R. D. Some normative data on the WAIS and its indices in an aged population. *Journal of Clinical Psychology,* 1966, *22*(2), 184–188.

Branconnier, R. J., & Cole, J. O. A memory assessment technique for use in geriatric psychopharmacology: Drug efficacy trial with naftifrofuryl. *Journal of the American Geriatrics Society,* 1977, *25*(4), 186–188.

Burnand, Y., Richard, J., Tissot, R., & de Ajuriaguerra, J. Nature of the operational deficit in the aged afflicted with degenerative dementia: Conservation of physical quantities, proofs of causality and transitivity. *Encephale,* 1972, *61,* 5–31.

Buschke, H., & Fuld, P. A. Evaluating storage, retention, and retrieval in disordered memory and learning. *Neurology,* 1974, *24*(11), 1019–1025.

Canter, A., & Straumanis, J. J. Performance of senile and healthy aged persons on the BIP Bender test. *Perceptual and Motor Skills,* 1969, *28*(3), 695–698.

Cantone, G., Orsini, A., Grossi, D., & De Michele, G. Verbal and spatial memory span in dementia (an experimental study of 185 subjects). *Acta Neurologia*(Napoli), 1978, *33*(2), 175–183.

Cox, J. R. Body water, electrolytes and psychological test performance in elderly patients. *Gerontologia Clinica,* 1973, *15*(4), 203–208.

Crookes, T. G. Indices of early dementia on WAIS. *Psychological Reports,* 1974, *34*(3), 734.

Diesfeldt, H. F. The distinction between long-term and short-term memory in senile dementia: An analysis of free recall and delayed recognition. *Neuropsychologia,* 1978, *16,* 115–119.

Gedye, J. L., Exton-Smith, A. N., & Wedgwood, J. A method for measuring mental performance in the elderly and its use in a pilot clinical trial of meclofenoxate in organic dementia (preliminary communication). *Age and Ageing,* 1972, *1*(2), 74–80.

Gordon, M. C. Some effects of stimulus presentation rate and complexity on perception and retention of brain-damaged patients. *Cortex,* 1970, *6*(3), 273–286.

Gottfries, C. G., Gottfries, I., & Roos, B. E. Homovanillic acid and 5-hydroxyindoleacetic acid in cerebrospinal fluid related to rated mental and motor impairment in senile and presenile dementia. *Acta Psychiatrica Scandinavica,* 1970, *46*(2), 99–105.

Hagberg, B. O., & Ingvar, D. H. Cognitive reduction in presenile dementia related to regional abnormalities of the cerebral blood flow. *British Journal of Psychiatry,* 1976, *128,* 209–222.

Hall, E. H., *et al.* Intellect, mental illness, and survival in the aged: A longitudinal investigation. *Journal of Gerontology,* 1972, *27*(2), 237–244.

Hemsi, L. K., Whitehead, A., & Post, F. Cognitive functioning and cerebral arousal in elderly depressives and dements. *Journal of Psychosomatic Research,* 1968, *12*(2), 145–156.

Hibbard, T. R., Migliaccio, J. N., Goldstone, S., & Lhamon, W. T. Temporal information processing by young and senior adults and patients with senile dementia. *Journal of Gerontology,* 1975, *30*(3), 326–330.

Hilbert, N. M., Niederehe, G., & Kahn, R. L. Accuracy and speed of memory in depressed and organic aged. *Educational Gerontology,* 1976, *1*(2), 131–146.

Hodkinson, H. M. Mental impairment in the elderly. *Journal of the Royal College of Physicians of London,* 1973, *7*(4), 305–317.

Hopkins, B., & Roth, M. Psychological test performance in patients over sixty. II. Paraphrenia, arteriosclerosis and acute confusion. *Journal of Mental Science,* 1953, *99,* 451–463.

Inglis, J. An experimental study of learning and memory function in elderly psychiatric patients. *Journal of Mental Science,* 1957, *103,* 796–803.

Inglis, J. Psychological investigations of cognitive deficit in elderly psychiatric patients. *Psychological Bulletin,* 1958, *55,* 197–214.

Jonsson, C. O., Edin, P., Soderberg, S., & Waldton, S. Exploratory behavior in patients suffering from senile dementia: A comparison with children. *Acta Psychiatrica Scandinavica,* 1976, *53*(4), 302–320.

Jonsson, C. O., Malhammar, G., & Waldton, S. Abnormalities in the orienting response in senile dementia. *Acta Psychiatrica Scandinavica,* 1976, *54*(5), 323–332.

Kempel, L. T. Orientation errors during successive administration of the Memory-for-Designs test. *Journal of Consulting and Clinical Psychology,* 1973, *4*(2), 314.

Kendrick, D. C., & Post, F. Differences in cognitive status between healthy, psychiatrically ill, and diffusely brain-damaged elderly subjects. *British Journal of Psychiatry,* 1967, *113,* 75–81.

Kettell, M. E. Perceptual and behavioral correlates of "organicity" in old age. *Journal of Geriatric Psychiatry,* 1976, *9,* 85–87.

Klingner, A., Ban, T. A., & Lehmann, H. E. Transference, discrimination and reversal: A comparison between normals and pathological groups. *Conditional Reflex,* 1972, *7*(4), 216–225.

Kramer, M., & Roth, T. Dreams and dementia: A laboratory exploration of dream recall and dream content in chronic brain syndrome patients. *International Journal of Aging and Human Development,* 1975, 6(2), 179–182.

Kramer, M., Roth, T., & Trinder, J. Dreams and dementia: A laboratory exploration of dream recall and dream content in chronic brain syndrome patients. *International Journal of Aging and Human Development,* 1975, 6(2), 169–178.

Larner, S. Encoding in senile dementia and elderly depressives: A preliminary study. *British Journal of Social and Clinical Psychology,* 1977, 16(4), 379–390.

Marksen, E. W., & Levitz, G. A Guttman scale to assess memory loss among the elderly. *Gerontologist,* 1973, 13(3), 337–340.

Miller, E. Efficiency of coding and the short-term memory defect in presenile dementia. *Neuropsychologia,* 1972, 10, 133–136.

Miller, E. Impaired recall and the memory disturbance in presenile dementia. *British Journal of Social and Clinical Psychology,* 1975, 14, 73–79.

Miller, E. On the nature of the memory disorder in presenile dementia. *Neuropsychologia,* 1971, 9, 75–81.

Miller, E. Psychomotor performance in presenile dementia. *Psychological Medicine,* 1974, 4, 65–68.

Miller, E. Retrieval from long-term memory in presenile dementia: Two tests of an hypothesis. *British Journal of Social and Clinical Psychology,* 1978, 17(2), 143–148.

Miller, E. Short- and long-term memory in patients with presenile dementia (Alzheimer's disease). *Psychological Medicine,* 1973, 3(2), 221–224.

Miller, E., & Lewis, P. Recognition memory in elderly patients with depression and dementia: A signal detection analysis. *Journal of Abnormal Psychology,* 1977, 86, 84–86.

Nelson, H. E. & McKenna, P. The use of current reading ability in the assessment of dementia. *British Journal of Social and Clinical Psychology,* 1975, *14*(3), 259–267.

Perez, F. I., Gay, J. R. & Taylor, R. L. WAIS performance of neurologically impaired aged. *Psychological Reports,* 1975, *37*(3), 1043–1047. (Part 2)

Perez, F. I., Gay, J. R., Taylor, R. L., & Rivera, V. M. Patterns of memory performance in the neurologically impaired aged. *Canadian Journal of Neurological Sciences,* 1975, *2*(4), 347–355.

Perez, F. I., Mathew, N. T., Stump, D. A., & Meyer, J. S. Regional cerebral blood flow: Statistical patterns and psychological performance in multi-infarct dementia and Alzheimer's disease. *Canadian Journal of Neurological Sciences,* 1977, *4*, 53–62.

Perez, F. I., Stump, D. A., Gay, J. R., & Hart, V. R. Intellectual performance in multi-infarct dementia and Alzheimer's disease: A replication study. *Canadian Journal of Neurological Sciences,* 1976, *3*(3), 181–187.

Perez, F., *et al.* Analysis of intellectual and cognitive performance in patients with multi-infarct dementia, vertebro-basilar insufficiency with dementia and Alzheimer's disease. *Journal of Neurology, Neurosurgery and Psychiatry,* 1975, *38*(6), 533–540.

Podnieks, I., & Doust, J. W. Spontaneous rhythms of perceptual motor performance in intact and damaged brain of man. *Biological Psychology,* 1975, *3*(3), 201–212.

Post, F. Disturbances of memory and thinking. *Gerontologist,* 1970, *10*, 5–8.

Shapiro, M. B., Post, F., Loefving, B., & Inglis, J. Memory function in psychiatric patients over 60: Some methodological and diagnostic implications. *Journal of Mental Science,* 1956, *106*, 233–246.

Solyom, L., & Barik, H. C. Conditioning in senescence and senility. *Journal of Gerontology,* 1965, *20*(4), 483–488.

Stonier, P. D. Score changes following repeated administration of mental status questionnaires. *Age and Ageing,* 1974, *3*(2), 291–296.

Tissot, R. Dementia and memory. *Encephale,* 1973, 62(6), 491–505.

Whitehead, A. Changes in cognitive functioning in elderly psychiatric patients. *British Journal of Psychiatry,* 1977, *130,* 605–608.

Whitehead, A. Recognition memory in dementia. *British Journal of Social and Clinical Psychology,* 1975, *14*(2), 191–194.

B. PSYCHOPHYSIOLOGICAL ASPECTS

Bower, H. M., Andrews, J. T., & Pope, R. A. Dementia and cerebral blood flow. *Medical Journal of Australia,* 1970, *1*(5), 207–211.

Butler, R. N., Dastur, D. K., & Perlin, S. Relationships of senile manifestations and chronic brain syndrome to cerebral circulation and metabolism. *Journal of Psychiatric Research,* 1965, *3*(4), 229–238.

Cahan, R. B., & Yeager, C. L. Admission EEG as a predictor of mortality and discharge for aged state hospital patients. *Journal of Gerontology,* 1966, *21*(2), 248–256.

Dascalov, D. EEG findings in Alzheimer's disease. *Electroencephalography and Clinical Neurophysiology,* 1969, *27*(4), 447.

De Risio, C., Urbani, M., & Ridolo, P. The orienting reflex in senile dementia. *Rivista di Neurologia,* 1966, *12*(4), 589–595.

Dekoninck, W. J., Calay, R., & Hongne, J. C. CBF in elderly with chronic cerebral involvement. *Acta Neurologica Scandinavica,* 1977, *56*(64), 412–413. (Supplement)

Editorial: Cerebral blood flow in dementia. *British Medical Journal,* 1976, *1*(6024), 1487–1488.

Ehle, A. L., & Johnson, P. C. Rapidly evolving EEG changes in a case of Alzheimer disease. *Annals of Neurology,* 1977, *1*(6), 593–595.

Gordon, E. B. Serial EEG studies in presenile dementia. *British Journal of Psychiatry,* 1968, *114*(511), 779–780.

Gustafson, L., & Risberg, J. Regional cerebral blood flow related to psychiatric symptoms in dementia with onset in the presenile period. *Acta Psychiatrica Scandinavica,* 1974, *50*(5), 516–538.

Gustafson, L., Hagberg, B., Holley, J. W., Risberg, J., & Ingvar, D. H. Regional cerebral blood flow in organic dementia with early onset. Correlations with psychiatric symptoms and psychometric variables. *Acta Neurologica Scandinavica,* 1970, *46,* (Supplement 43:74–75).

Gustafson, L., Risberg, J., Hagberg, B., Hougaard, K., Nilsson, L., & Ingvar, D. H. Cerebral blood flow, EEG and psychometric variables related to clinical findings in presenile dementia. *Acta Neurologica Scandinavica,* 1972, *51,* 439–440. (Supplement)

Hachinski, V., Iliff, L., Zilhka, E., Boulay, G., McAllister, V., Marshall, J., Russell, R., & Symon, L. Cerebral blood flow in dementia. *Archives of Neurology,* 1975, *32*(9), 632–637.

Hagberg, B. Defects of immediate memory related to the cerebral blood flow distribution. *Brain and Language,* 1978, *5*(3), 366–367.

Hagberg, B. O., & Ingvar, D. H. Cognitive reduction in presenile dementia related to regional abnormalities of the cerebral blood flow. *British Journal of Psychiatry,* 1976, *128,* 209–222.

Hoyer, S., Oesterreich, K., Weinhardt, F., & Kruger, G. Blood flow and oxidative metabolism of the brain in patients with dementia (author's translation). *Journal of Neurology* (Ger), 1975, *210*(4), 227–237.

Ingvar, D. H. Regional cerebral blood flow in organic dementia and in chronic schizophrenia. *Triangle,* 1974, *13,* 17–23.

Ingvar, D. H., & Gustafson, L. Regional cerebral blood flow in organic dementia with early onset. *Acta Neurologica Scandinavica,* 1970, *46,* (Supplement 43:42 +).

Ingvar, D. H., Risberg, J., & Schwartz, M. S. Evidence of subnormal function of association cortex in presenile dementia. *Neurology,* 1975, *25*(10), 964–974.

Ingvar, D., *et al.* General and regional abnormalities of cerebral blood flow in senile and presenile dementia. *Scandinavian Journal of Clinical and Laboratory Investigation,* 1968, *102,* 12B. (Supplement 22)

Johannesson, G., Brun, A., Gustafson, I., & Ingvar, D. H. EEG in presenile dementia related to cerebral blood flow and autopsy findings. *Acta Neurologica Scandinavica,* 1977, *56*(2), 89–103.

Kajiwara, A. Electroencephalographic studies on cerebral diseases in presenium and senium. *Psychiatria et Neurologia Japonica,* 1968, *70*(4), 277–301.

Kanowski, S. EEG and geriatric psychiatry. *Brain,* 1971, *30*(3), 268.

Lars, G. Emotional behaviour, personality changes and cognitive reduction in presenile dementia: Related to regional cerebral blood flow. *Acta Psychiatrica Scandinavica,* 1975, *257,* 39–71. (Supplement)

Levy, R., Isaacs, A., & Behrman, J. Neurophysiological correlates of senile dementia. II. The somatosensory evoked response. *Psychological Medicine,* 1971, *1*(2), 159–165.

Lorizio, A. On abnormalities of spindle waves in sleep in senile dementia. *Rivista di Neurologia,* 1966, *12*(4), 655–660.

Morozova, T. V. Correlational analysis of the frequency of alpha rhythms in the EEG of healthy middle-age people and patients with senile psychoses. *Zhurnal Nevropatologii i Psikhiatrii,* 1970, *70*(11), 1667–1671.

Morozova, T. V. Spatial synchronization of alpha-activity in the cerebral cortex in patients with psychoses in advanced age. *Zhurnal Nevropatologii i Psikhiatrii,* 1967, *67*(4), 560–567.

Muller, H. F. Generalized sharp activity in the electroencephalogram of middle-aged and elderly psychiatric patients. *Journal of the American Geriatrics Society,* 1969, *17*(4), 337–359.

Muller, H. F., & Grad, B. Clinical-psychological, electroencephalographic and adrenocortical relationships in elderly psychiatric patients. *Journal of Gerontology,* 1974, *29,* 28–38.

Obrist, W. D. Electroencephalography in aging and dementia. In R. Katzman & R. Terry (Eds.), *Alzheimer's Disease, Senile Dementia, and Related Disorders.* New York: Raven Press, in press.

Obrist, W. D., Chivian, E., Cronqvist, S., & Ingvar, D. H. Regional cerebral blood flow in senile and presenile dementia. *Neurology*(Minneapolis), 1970, *20*(4), 315–322.

Olesen, J., Simard, D., Paulson, O., & Skinhoj, E. Focal cerebral blood flow, reactivity of cerebral blood vessels and cerebral oxydative metabolism in certain groups of patients with organic dementia. *Acta Neurologica Scandinavica,* 1970, *46,* (Supplement 43:76).

Oliveros, J. C. EEG in organic psychosis. *Electroencephalography and Clinical Neurophysiology,* 1970, *29,* 99.

Perez, F. I., Mathew, N. T., Stump, D. A., & Meyer, J. S. Regional cerebral blood flow statistical patterns and psychological performance in multi-infarct dementia and Alzheimer's disease. *Canadian Journal of Neurological Sciences,* 1977, *4,* 53–62.

Roman, I. Proceedings: Some particular EEG aspects in dementia. *Electroencephalography and Clinical Neurophysiology,* 1975, *39*(5), 535.

Short, M. J., Musella, L., & Wilson, W. P. Correlation of affect and EEG in senile psychoses. *Journal of Gerontology,* 1968, *23*(3), 324–327.

Simard, D., Olesen, J., Paulson, O. B., Lassen, N. A., & Skinhof, E. Regional cerebral blood flow and its regulation in dementia. *Brain,* 1971, *94*(2), 273–288.

Stefoski, D., Bergen, D., Fox, J., Morrell, F., Huckman, M., & Ramsey, R. Correlation between diffuse EEG abnormalities and cerebral atrophy in senile dementia. *Journal of Neurology, Neurosurgery, and Psychiatry,* 1976, *39*(8), 751–755.

Stensman, R., & Ingvar, D. H. EEG and cerebral circulation in pre-senile dementia. *Electroencephalography and Clinical Neurophysiology,* 1971, *30*(3), 268.

Surwillo, W. W. Timing of behavior in senescence and the role of the central nervous system. In G. A. Talland (Ed.), *Human Aging and Behavior.* New York: Academic Press, 1968.

Thompson, L. W., & Marsh, G. R. Psychophysiological studies of aging. In C. Eisdorfer & M. P. Lawton (Eds.), *The Psychology of Adult Development and Aging.* Washington, D.C.: American Psychological Association, 1973.

Visser, S. L., Stam, F. C., van Tilburg, W., den Velde, W., Blom, J. L., & de Rijke, W. Visual evoked response in senile and presenile dementia. *Electroencephalography and Clinical Neurophysiology,* 1976, *40*(4), 385–392.

Wang, H. S., Obrist, W. D., & Busse, E. W. Neurophysiological correlates of the intellectual function. In E. Palmore (Ed.), *Normal Aging II.* Durham, N. C.: Duke University, 1974.

Wilson, W. P., Musella, L., & Short, M. J. The electroencephalogram in dementia. *Contemporary Neurology Series,* 1977, *15,* 205–221.

C. OTHER BEHAVIORAL MANIFESTATIONS

Adams, R. D. Recent observations on normal pressure hydrocephalus. *Schweizer Archive fur Neurologie, Neurochirurgie und Psychiatrie,* 1975, *116,* 7–15.

Aggernaes, A., & Myscheitzky, A. Experienced reality in somatic patients more than 65 years old. A comparative study of disturbed and clear, but demented states of consciousness. *Acta Psychiatrica Scandinavica,* 1976, *54*(4), 225–237.

Amand, G. Absence states and prolonged states of confusion after the age of 60 years. *Rev. Electroencephalogr. Neurophysiol. Clin.*(Fr.), 1976, *1*(2), 221–223.

Anderson, J. F. A study of disturbed behaviour in patients with dementia in two hospital populations. *Gerontologia Clinica,* 1970, *12,* 49–64.

Barshtein, E. I. Clinical features of the initial stages of senile dementive processes. *Zhurnal Nevropatologii i Psikhiatrii,* 1968, *68*(8), 1204–1209.

Beresewicz, M. Clinical picture of mental disorders in myxedema. *Psychiatria Polska,* 1978, *12,* 95–98.

Bettner, L. G., & Blum, J. E. Kent-Rosanoff Free Association Test in aged twins with and without organic brain syndrome. *Proceedings of the American Psychological Association,* 1972, *7,* 651–652.

Black, F. W., & Strub, R. L. Behavioral disorders reflecting organic disease (letter). *New England Journal of Medicine,* 1975, *292*(19), 1029.

Blessed, G., Tomlinson, B. E., & Roth, M. The association between quantitative measures of dementia and of senile change in the cerebral grey matter of elderly subjects. *British Journal of Psychiatry,* 1968, *114*(512), 797–811.

Buchan, T. Organic confusional states. *South African Medical Journal,* 1972, *46*(37), 1340–1343.

Cameroń, O. E. Studies in senile nocturnal delusion. *Psychiatric Quarterly,* 1941, *15,* 47–53.

Cazzullo, C. L. Psychological aspects of cerebral arteriosclerosis. *Foreign Psychiatry,* 1972, *1*(3), 231–238.

Cox, J. R., & Orme, J. E. Body water, electrolytes and psychological test performance in elderly patients. *Gerontologia Clinica,* 1973, *15*(4), 203–208.

Crowell, R. M., Tew, J. M., & Mark, V. H. Aggressive dementia associated with normal pressure hydrocephalus: Report of two unusual cases. *Neurology,* 1973, *23*(5), 461–464.

Davies, G., Hamilton, S., Hendrickson, D. E., Levy, R., & Post, F. Psychological test performance and sedation thresholds of elderly dements, depressives and depressives with incipient brain damage. *Psychological Medicine,* 1978, *8,* 103–109.

de Ajuriaguerra, J., & Tissot, R. Some aspects of psycho-neurological disintegration in senile dementia. In C. Muller & L. Ciompi (Eds.), *Senile Dementia.* Bern: Hans Huber, 1968.

de Ajuriaguerra, J., *et al.* Disintegration of the elements of time in the degenerative dementias of old age. *Encephale,* 1967, *56,* 385–438.

de Ajuriaguerra, J., Richard, J., Tissot, R., Vengos, P., Luke, A., & Raboud, A. M. Eating behavior in degenerative dementias or mixed dementias with a predominance of degeneration in old age. *Annales Medico-Psychologiques,* 1976, *2*(2), 214–241.

DeJong, R. N. The neurologic aspects of dementia. *Transactions of the American Neurological Association,* 1973, *98,* 109–113.

Dekoninck, W. J., Collard, M., & Noel, G. Cerebral vasoreactivity in senile dementia. *Gerontology,* 1977, *23*(2), 148–160.

Delwaide, P. J., Devoitille, M., & Ylieff, M. The clinical picture of cerebral senility. *Revue Medicale de Liege*(Fre.), 1976, *31*(23), 711–719.

Ernst, P., Badash, D., Beran, B., Kosovsky, R., & Kleinhauz, M. Incidence of mental illness in the aged: Unmasking the effects of a diagnosis of chronic brain syndrome. *Journal of the American Geriatrics Society,* 1977, *25*(8), 371–375.

Fot, K., Richard, J., Tissot, R., & de Ajuriaguerra, J. The extinction phenomenon in simultaneous tactile stimulation of the face and hand in senile degenerative dementia. *Neuropsychologia,* 1970, *8*(4), 493–500.

Gaillard, J. M. The disintegration of the body schema in elderly patients with states of dementia. *Journal de Psychologie Normale et Pathologique,* 1970, *4,* 443–472.

Gainotti, G., Confabulation of denial in senile dementia. An experimental study. *Psychiatrica Clinica,* 1975, *8*(3), 99–108.

Gainotti, G. Disintegration and reorganization of behavior in dementia. *Archivio di Psicologia Neurologia y Psichiatria,* 1971, *32*(5), 443–466.

Gainotti, G. Intellectual deterioration and psycho-motor disintegration in dementia. *Acta Neurologica,* 1970, *25,* 607–627.

Goldstein, G., & Shelly, C. H. Similarities and differences between psychological deficit in aging and brain damage. *Journal of Gerontology,* 1975, *30,* 448–455.

Goodwin, D. W., Alderson, P., & Rosenthal, R. Clinical significance of hallucinations in psychiatric disorders. A study of 116 hallucinatory patients. *Archives of General Psychiatry,* 1971, *24,* 76–80.

Gustafson, L. Psychiatric symptoms in dementia with onset in the presenile period. *Acta Psychiatrica Scandinavica,* 1975, *257,* 7–35. (Supplement)

Gustafson, L., & Hagberg, B. Dementia with onset in the presenile period. A cross-sectional study. *Acta Psychiatrica Scandinavica,* 1975, *257,* 3–71. (Supplement)

Gustafson, L., & Risberg, J. Regional cerebral blood flow related to psychiatric symptoms in dementia with onset in the presenile period. *Acta Psychiatrica Scandinavica,* 1974, *50*(5), 516–538.

Gustafson, L., Hagberg, B., & Ingvar, D. H. Speech disturbances in presenile dementia related to local cerebral blood flow abnormalities in the dominant hemisphere. *Brain and Language,* 1978, *5,* 103–118.

Haglund, R. M., & Schuckit, M. A., A clinical comparison of tests of organicity in elderly patients. *Journal of Gerontology,* 1976, *31*(6), 654–659.

Hattangadi, S. B., Grad, B., Beckett, M. E., & Csank, J. Z. Some clinical and biochemical variables in patients with chronic brain syndrome. *Journal of the American Geriatrics Society,* 1973, *21*(10), 460–464.

Heidell, E. D., & Kidd, A. H. Depression and senility. *Journal of Clinical Psychology,* 1975, *31*(4), 643–645.

Hopkins, B., & Roth, M. Psychological test performance in patients over sixty. II. Paraphrenics, arteriosclerotic psychosis and acute confusion. *Journal of Mental Science,* 1953, *99,* 451–463.

Jarema, M., & Wdowiak, L. EEG in the evaluation of symptoms in organic brain lesions. *Psychiatra Polska,* 1977, *11*(4), 437–444.

Joannides, A. A. Visual perceptual activity in degenerative dementia of old age. *Cortex,* 1971, *7*(3), 292–316.

Jonsson, C. O., Edin, P., Soderberg, S., & Waldton, S. Exploratory behavior in patients suffering from senile dementia: A comparison with children. *Acta Psychiatrica Scandinavica,* 1976, *53*(4), 302–320.

Jonsson, C. O., Malhammar, G., & Waldton, S. Abnormalities in the orienting response in senile dementia. *Acta Psychiatrica Scandinavica,* 1976, *54*(5), 323–332.

Jonsson, C. O., Waldton, S., & Malhammar, G. The psychiatric symptomatology in senile dementia assessed by means of an interview. *Acta Psychiatrica Scandinavica,* 1972, *48*(2), 103–121.

Jonsson, C., Malhammar, G., & Waldton, S. Reflex elecitation thresholds in senile dementia. *Acta Psychiatrica Scandinavica,* 1977, *55*(2), 81–96.

Kahn, R. L., Zarit, S. H., Hilbert, N. M., & Niederehe, G. Memory complaint and impairment in the aged. The effect of depression and altered brain function. *Archives of General Psychiatry,* 1975, *32*(12), 1569–1573.

Krassoievitch, M., Weber, K., & Junod, J. P. Disintegration of the sleep cycle in senile dementia. *Schweizer Archiv fuer Neurologie Neurochirurgie und Psychiatrie,* 1965, *96*, 170–179.

Langley, G. E. Confusion in the elderly (letter). *Lancet,* 1977, *1*(8006), 312–313.

Lars, G. Psychiatric symptoms in dementia with onset in the presenile period. *Acta Psychiatrica Scandinavica,* 1975, *257*, 9–35. (Supplement)

Lawson, I. R. Confusion in the house: The assessment of disorientation for the familiar in the home. *Psychiatric Quarterly,* 1969, *43*, 225–239.

Levy, R., Isaacs, A., & Behrman, J. Neurophysiological correlates of senile dementia. II. The somatosensory evoked response. *Psychological Medicine,* 1971, *1*(2), 159–165.

Lipowski, Z. J. Delirium, clouding of consciousness and confusion. *The Journal of Nervous and Mental Disease,* 1967, *145*(3), 227–255.

Liston, B. H. Occult presenile dementia. *Journal of Nervous and Mental Disease,* 1977, *164*(4), 263–267.

Macmillan, D., & Shaw, P. Senile breakdown in standards of personal and environmental cleanliness. *British Medical Journal,* 1966, *2*(521), 1032–1037.

McDonald, C. Clinical heterogeneity in senile dementia. *British Journal of Psychiatry,* 1969, *115*(520), 267–271.

Murley, H. D., Milam, D. R., & Gorman, W. Objective psychiatric and psychologic signs of brain disorders. *Arizona Medicine,* 1976, *33*(11), 891–895.

Murphy, E. The confused elderly patient. *Journal of the Irish Medical Association,* 1968, *61*(369), 99–103.

O'Brien, M. D. Some neurological aspects of dementia. *Gerontologia Clinica* (Basel), 1971, *13*(6), 339–349.

Overall, J. E., & Gorham, D. R. Organicity versus old age in objective and projective test performance. *Journal of Consulting and Cinical Psychology,* 1972, *39,* 98–105.

Parkes, J. D., *et al.* Parkinson's disease, cerebral arteriosclerosis, and senile dementia. Clinical features and response to levodopa. *Quarterly Journal of Medicine,* 1974, *43*(169), 49–61.

Perrot, E., de. The family of the aged schizophrenic and the senile dementia case in relation to the patient. *Encephale,* 1964, *53*(3), 383–404.

Peterson, G. C. Psychiatric aspects of chronic organic brain syndrome. *Postgraduate Medicine,* 1976, *60*(5), 162–168.

Pitt, B. The muddled patient. *Practitioner,* 1978, *220*(1316), 199–202.

Plutachik, R., & Discipio, W. J. Personality patterns in chronic alcoholism (Korsakoff's Syndrome), chronic schizophrenia, and geriatric patients with chronic brain syndrome. *Journal of the American Geriatrics Society,* 1974, *22*(11), 514–516.

Poser, C. M. The presenile dementias. *Journal of the American Medical Association,* 1975, *233,* 81–84.

Postel, J. Difficulty in recognizing oneself in the mirror in late dementia. *Evolution Psychiatrique,* 1968, *33,* 605–648.

Price, T. R. & Tucker, G. J. Psychiatric and behavioral manifestations of normal pressure hydrocephalus: A case report and brief review. *Journal of Nervous and Mental Disease,* 1977, *164,* 51–55.

Reed, H. B. C., Jr., & Reitan, R. M. A comparison of the effects of the normal aging process with the effects of organic brain damage on adaptive abilities. *Journal of Gerontology,* 1963, *18,* 177–179.

Reitan, R. M. The comparative psychological significance of aging in groups with and without organic brain damage. In C. Tibbitts & W. Donahue (Eds.), *Social and Psychological Aspects of Aging.* New York: Columbia University Press, 1962.

Reitan, R. M. Problems and prospects in studying the psychological correlates of brain lesions. *Cortex,* 1966, *2,* 127–154.

Reitan, R. M. Psychologic changes associated with aging and with cerebral damage. *Mayo Clinic Proceedings,* 1967, *42,* 653–673.

Rice, E. Organic brain syndromes and suicide. *International Journal of Psychoanalytic Psychotherapy,* 1973, *2*(3), 338–363.

Rochford, G. A study of naming errors in dysphasic and in demented patients. *Neuropsychologia,* 1971, *9*(4), 437–443.

Rosin, A. H. The physical and behavioural complex of dementia. *Gerontology,* 1977, *23,* 37–46.

Roth, M. Cerebral disease and mental disorders of old age as causes of antisocial behavior. *Int. Psychiatry Clin.,* 1968, *5*(3), 35–58.

Savitsky, E., & Sharkey, H. The geriatric patient and his family. Study of family interaction in the aged. *Journal of Geriatric Psychiatry,* 1972, *5,* 3–24.

Shahine, O., Rakhawy, Y. T., & Fawzy, A. Cerebral athero-sclerosis: A correlative study between physical and psychological pictures. *Journal of the Egyptian Medical Association,* 1970, *53*(6), 419–432.

Sherwin, I., & Seltzer, B. Senile and presenile dementia: A clinical overview. In K. Nandy & I. Sherwin (Eds.), *The Aging Brain and Senile Dementia.* New York: Plenum Press, 1977.

Shumskii, N. G. Clinical characteristics of some hallucinatory-delirious psychoses of old age. *Zhurnal Nevropatologii i Psikhiatrii,* 1974, *74*(2), 256–263.

Slater, R., & Lipman, A. Staff assessments of confusion and the situation of confused residents in homes for old people. *Gerontologist,* 1977, *17*(6), 523–530.

Sternberg, E. Psychotic, functional, early stages of senile mental disorders. *Psychiatrie Neurologie und Medizinische Psychologie,* 1972, *24*(6), 318–325.

Szobor, A. The role of intellectual decline and affectivity in crimes committed in old age. *Morphol. Igazsagugyi Orv. Sz.,* 1972, *12*(3), 202–208.

Trier, T. R. Characteristics of mentally ill aged: A comparison of patients with psychogenic disorders and patients with organic brain syndromes. *Journal of Gerontology,* 1966, *21*(3), 354–364.

Tupikov, A. M. Confabulation in atrophic and vascular disease of old age: Clinico-psychopathologic findings. *Zhurnal Nevropatologii i Psikhiatrii,* 1976, *76*(8), 1181–1186.

Weinberg, J. Understanding mentally confused elderly persons. *Postgraduate Medicine,* 1970, *47*(3), 116–119.

Wertheimer, J., & Mentenopoulos, G. Study of opto-kinetic nystagmus in aged persons with organic psychosis. Description of a method and its use in geronto-psychiatric environment. *Schweizer Archiv fuer Neurologie Neurochirurgie und Psychiatrie,* 1973, *112,* 155–175.

Wieck, H. H. Psychopathology of cerebrovascular processes. *Internist*(Berlin), 1976, *17,* 45–51.

Zarit, S. H., & Kahn, R. L. Aging and adaptation to illness. *Journal of Gerontology,* 1975, *30, 67–72.*

Zarit, S. H., & Kahn, R. L. Impairment and adaptation in chronic disabilities: Spatial inattention. *Journal of Nervous and Mental Disease,* 1974, *159,* 63–72.

IV. ACUTE ORGANIC BRAIN SYNDROME

Abrahamson, I. A., Sr., & Abrahamson, I. A., Jr. Dehydration: A cause of psychosis following cataract extraction. *Eye, Ear, Nose and Throat Monthly,* 1968, *47*(3), 144–146.

Adams, P. E. Pharmacologic management of psychiatric emergencies. *Pennsylvania Medicine,* 1977, *80*(2), 49–52.

Aderhold, R. M., & Muniz, C. E. Acute psychosis with amitriptyline and furazolidone. *Journal of the American Medical Association,* 1970, *213*(12), 2080.

Agulnik, P. L., Dimascio, A., & Moore, P. Acute brain syndrome associated with lithium therapy. *American Journal of Psychiatry,* 1972, *129*(5), 621–623.

Ananth, J. V., Ban, T. A., & Lehmann, H. E. Toxic psychotic syndrome associated with chlorpromazine administration. *Canadian Medical Association Journal,* 1970, *102*(6), 642.

Anwar, M. Letter: Digoxin and confusion in the elderly. *British Medical Journal,* 1975, *3*(5977), 231.

Are there any reports of organic brain syndrome resulting from concomitant use of phenothiazines and anti-Parkinsonian agents? *New York State Journal of Medicine,* 1973, *73*(24), 2898–2899.

Baile, W. F., De Paulo, J. R., & Schmidt, C. W. Emergency room management of organic brain syndromes caused by over-the-counter hypnotics. *Maryland State Medical Journal,* 1977, *26,* 61–63.

Brion, S., & Guerin, R. Drug-induced mental confusion during chemotherapy of psychiatric diseases. Possible role of trihexyphenidyl. *Therapie,* 1975, *30*(3), 447-450.

Carney, M. W. Bromism: A clinical chameleon. *Nursing Times,* 1973, *69*(27), 859-861.

Clower, C. G., Young, A. J., & Kepas, D. Psychotic states resulting from disorders of thyroid function. *Johns Hopkins Medical Journal,* 1969, *124*(6), 305-310.

Cohen, S. I. Letter: Recoverable organic psychosis after hypopituitary coma. *British Medical Journal,* 1976, *1*(6013), 831.

Cordeiro, J. D. Late delirious states. Hereditary, biotype, premorbid personality. *Evolutionary Psychiatry,* 1972, *37*(2), 331-347.

Cunningham, T. A. Letter: Adverse reaction to flurazepam. *Canadian Medical Association Journal,* 1975, *112*(7), 805.

De Beer, J. M., & Simons, C. H. Psychopharmaceuticals as cause of pseudo-dementia. *Nederlands Tijdschrift voor Geneeskunde,* 1977, *121*(16), 664-666.

Delaney, J. C., & Ravey, M. Cimetidine and mental confusion (letter). *Lancet,* 1977, *2*(8036), 512.

Devaul, R. A. Acute organic brain syndromes: Clinical considerations. *Texas Medicine,* 1976, *72*(2), 51-54.

Devaul, R. A., & Zisook, S. Reversible organic brain syndrome: Clues to quick recognition. *Medical Times,* 1977, *105*(8), (80)9D.

Drtil, J. Psychotic syndromes after long term use of analgesics: Antipyretics. *Act. Nerv. Super.,* 1972, *14*(3), 186-187.

Eraut, D. Idiopathic hypoparathyroidism presenting as dementia. *British Medical Journal,* 1974, *1*(905), 429-430.

Fox, J. H., Topel, J. L., & Huckman, M. S. Dementia in the elderly: A search for treatable illnesses. *Journal of Gerontology,* 1975, *30*(5), 557-564.

Fraser, H. S., & Carr, A. C. Propranolol psychosis (letter). *British Journal of Psychiatry,* 1976, *129,* 508–509.

Freemon, F. R. Evaluation of patients with progressive intellectual deterioration. *Archives of Neurology,* 1976, *33*(9), 658–659.

Furhoff, A. K. Adverse mental effects of beta blockaders. *Lakartidningen,* 1976, *73*(45), 3909.

Gaedt, C., & Helmchen, H. Problems of mental side effects of drugs. *Hippokrates,* 1970, *41*(4), 431–452.

Gilbert, G. J. Quinidine dementia. *American Journal of Cardiology,* 1978, *41*(4), 791.

Grant, I., & Judd, L. L. Neuropsychological and EEG disturbances in polydrug users. *American Journal of Psychiatry,* 1976, *133*(9), 1039–1042.

Gupta, V. P., & Ehrlich, G. E. Organic brain syndrome in rheumatoid arthritis following corticosteroid withdrawal. *Arthritis and Rheumatism,* 1976, *19*(6), 1333–1338.

Hart, R. J., & McCurdy, P. R. Psychosis in vitamin B 12 deficiency. *Archives of Internal Medicine,* 1971, *128*(4), 596–597.

Hawkins, D. J. Acute organic brain syndrome psychosis with methyldopa therapy: Case report. *Missouri Medicine,* 1976, *73*(8), 476; 481.

Helmchen, H., & Hippius, H. Exogenous reaction types and psychiatric pharmacotherapy. *Deutsch Medical Journal,* 1968, *19*(9), 299–304.

Hendrickx, J. Reversible confusional states in the aged. *Tijdschrift voor Sociale Geneeskunde,* 1969, *25,* 195–200.

Herridge, C. F., & Brooke, M. F. Ephedrine psychosis. *British Medical Journal,* 1968, *2*(598), 160.

Hosek, K. Acute gerontopsychiatric states in catamnesis. *Ceskoslovenska Psychiatrie,* 1977, *73*(5), 316–320.

Hughes, C. P., Myers, F. K., Smith, K., & Libow, L. S. Pseudo-senility: Acute and reversible organic brain syndromes. *Journal of the American Geriatrics Society,* 1973, *21*(3), 112–120.

Jacobs, L. S., Green, R. A., Gillin, J. C., & Wyatt, R. J. Phenelzine and psychosis. *Hawaii Medical Journal,* 1976, *35*(4), 109–111.

Jana, D. K., & Romano-Jana, L. Hypernatremic psychosis in the elderly: Case reports. *Journal of the American Geriatrics Society,* 1973, *21*(10), 473–477.

Katz, N. M., Agle, D. P., DePalma, R. G., & De Cosse, J. J. Delirium in surgical patients under intensive care. *Archives of Surgery,* 1972, *104,* 310–313.

Kendel, K., & Fodor, S. Pulmonary embolism and symptomatic psychosis. *Deutsche Medizinische Wochenschrift,* 1968, *93*(25), 1238–1241.

Knee, S. T., & Razani, J. Acute organic brain syndrome: A complication of disulfiram therapy. *American Journal of Psychiatry,* 1974, *131*(11), 1281–1282.

Langley, G. E. Confusion in the elderly. *Lancet,* 1977, *1*(8006), 312–313.

Libow, L. S. Senile dementia and "pseudosenility": Clinical diagnosis. In C. Eisdorfer & F. O. Friedel (Eds.), *Cognitive and Emotional Disturbance in the Elderly.* New York: Plenum, 1977.

Libow, L. S. Pseudo-senility: Acute and reversible organic brain syndromes. *Journal of the American Geriatrics Society,* 1973, *21*(3), 112–120.

Linn, L., Kahn, R. L., Coles, R., Cohen, J., Marshall, D., & Weinstein, E. A. Behavior disturbances following cataract extraction. *American Journal of Psychiatry,* 1953, *110,* 281–289.

Maruta, T. Prescription drug-induced organic brain syndrome. *American Journal of Psychiatry,* 1978, *135*(3), 376–377.

McMillen, M. A., Ambis, D., & Siegel, J. H. Cimetidine and mental confusion (letter). *New England Journal of Medicine,* 1978, *298*(5), 284–285.

Nicol, C. F. Treatment of reversible dementia. *New York State Journal of Medicine,* 1970, *70*(19), 2432–2437.

Nyland, H. Ephedrine, abuse and psychosis. *Tidsskrift for den Norske Laegeforening,* 1973, *93*(27), 2027–2029.

O'Connel, G., Campbell, P., & Anath, J. Amitriptyline: Initial intolerance and subsequent psychosis. *Canadian Medical Association Journal,* 1972, *106*(2), 115.

Ochitill, H. N., & Amberson, J. Acute cerebral symptomatology, a rare presentation of scleromyxedema. *Journal of Clinical Psychiatry,* 1978, *39*(5), 471–475.

Padfield, P. L., Smith, D. A., Fitzsimons, E. J., & McCruden, D. C. Disopyramide and acute psychosis (letter). *Lancet,* 1977, *1*(8022), 1152.

Parker, B., Deibler, S., Feldshuh, B., Frosch, W., Laureano, E., & Sillen, J. Finding medical reasons for psychiatric behavior. *Geriatrics,* 1976, *31*(6), 87–91.

Raskind, M. A., Kitchell, M., & Alvarez, C. Bromide intoxication in the elderly. *Journal of the American Geriatrics Society,* 1978, *26*(5), 222–224.

Reilly, P. P. Anticholinergic toxicity. Disorder manifested by confusion and delirium results when two or more medications with side effects are given. *Rhode Island Medical Journal,* 1977, *60*(6), 293–296.

Robinson, T. J., & Mulligan, T. O. Cimetidine and mental confusion (letter). *Lancet,* 1977, *2*(8040), 719.

Roder, E. Reversible psychosis and dementia in myxedema. *Acta Psychiatrica Scandinavica,* 1970, *46*, 1–13.

Roder, E., & Olivarius, B. The reversible organic psychosyndrome in hypothyroidism. *Acta Neurologia Scandinavica,* 1970, *46*, (Supplement 43:81–82).

Rudd, T. N. Prescribing methods and iatrogenic situations in old age. *Gerontologia Clinica,* 1972, *14*(2), 123–128.

Saker, B., Musk, A., Haywood, E., & Hurst, P. Reversible toxic psychosis after cephalexin. *Medical Journal of Australia,* 1973, *1*(10), 497–498.

Shulman, R. A survey of vitamin B12 deficiency in an elderly psychiatric population. *British Journal of Psychiatry,* 1967, *113,* 449–471.

Simon, A., & Cahan, R. The acute brain syndrome in geriatric patients. In W. M. Mendel, & L. J. Epstein (Eds.), *Acute Psychotic Reaction.* Washington, D. C.: Psychiatric Research Reports of the American Medical Psychiatric Association, 1963.

Sprints, A. M., & Shenderov, B. L. On psychoses caused by asthmatol. *Zhurnal Nevropatologii i Psikhiatrii,* 1968, *68*(3), 431–436.

Stonecypher, D. D. The cause and prevention of postoperative psychoses in the elderly. *American Journal of Ophthalmology,* 1963, *55,* 605–610.

Stork-Groenveld, I., & Meerloo, J. A. Acute mental confusion in elderly. *Praxis,* 1971, *60*(25), 844–847.

Thornton, W. E. Dementia induced by methyldopa with haloperidol. *New England Journal of Medicine,* 1976, *294*(22), 1222.

Topliss, D., & Bond, R. Acute brain syndrome after propranolol treatment (letter). *Lancet,* 1977, *2*(8048), 1133–1134.

von Tiggelen, C. J. Acute confusional states in the elderly (author's translation). *Aktuelle Gerontologie,* 1977, *7*(9), 499–502.

Wahl, C., Golden, J., Liston, E., Rimer, D., Rose, A., Soghor, D., & Solomon, D. Toxic and functional psychoses. Diagnosis and treatment in a medical setting. *Annals of Internal Medicine,* 1967, *66*(59), 989–1007.

Williams, R. J. Organic psychosis: Letter. *British Medical Journal,* 1974, *3*(5931), 629.

Young, J. P. Acute psychiatric disturbances in the elderly and their treatment. *British Journal of Clinical Practitioners,* 1972, *26*(11), 513–516.

Yvonneau, M., Aretche, N., & Leroy, S. Acute senile delirium. *Encephale,* 1973, 62(4), 367–381.

V. DIAGNOSIS AND ASSESSMENT

Aita, J. A., Senile dementia check list. To be considered before sending patients to nursing homes. *Nebraska Medical Journal,* 1971, *56*(11), 435–437.

Alexander, D. A. The application of the Graham-Kendall memory-for-designs test to elderly normal and psychiatric groups. *British Journal of Social and Clinical Psychology,* 1970, *9,* 85–86.

Alexander, D. A. Two tests of psychomotor function in detection of organic cerebral damage in elderly psychiatric patients. *Perceptual and Motor Skills,* 1971, *33,* 1291–1297.

Ames, L. B. Calibration of aging. *Journal of Personality Assessment,* 1974, *38*(6), 507–529.

Angel, R. W. Understanding and diagnosing senile dementia. *Geriatrics,* 1977, *32*(8), 47–49.

Arie, T. Dementia in the elderly: Diagnosis and assessment. *British Medical Journal,* 1973, *4*(891), 540–543.

Babcock, H. An experiment in the measurement of mental deterioration. *Archives of Psychology,* 1930, *18,* 5–105.

Bannister, R., Gilford, E., & Kocen, R. Isotope encephalography in the diagnosis of dementia due to communicating hydrocephalus. *Lancet,* 1967, *2*(524), 1014–1017.

Barnes, G. W., & Lucas, G. J. Cerebral dysfunction vs. psychogenesis in Halstead-Reitan tests. *Journal of Nervous and Mental Disease*, 1974, *158*(1), 50–60.

Barrett, E. T., Jr., & Logue, P. E. The use of the spiral after-effect test to differentiate chronic schizophrenics from chronic organics. *Journal of Clinical Psychology*, 1974, *30*(4), 513–516.

Bender, A. L., & Van Allen, M. W. Aspects of neuropsychological assessment with cerebral disease. In C. M. Gaitz (Ed.), *Aging and the Brain*. New York: Plenum, 1972.

Berzewski, H., & Selbach, H. Neuropsychiatric geriatrics: Diagnostics and therapy. *Internist* (Berlin), 1970, *11*(7), 244–250.

Birkett, D. P. The psychiatric differentiation of senility and arteriosclerosis. *British Journal of Psychiatry,* 1972, *120*(556), 321–325.

Blum, J. E., & Jarvik, L. F. Variations in intellectual decline as indicators of pathology: A longitudinal twin study. *Proceedings of the American Psychological Association,* 1969, *77*, 743–744.

Botwinick, J., & Birren, J. E. Differential decline in the Wechsler-Bellevue subtest in the senile psychoses. *Journal of Gerontology*, 1951, *6*, 365–368.

Bower, H. M. The differential diagnosis of dementia. *Medical Journal of Australia*, 1971, *2*(12), 623–626.

Brahm, J., Sarova-Pinhas, I., Front, D., & Goldhammer, Y. A simple CSF manometric test for adult hydrocephalus associated with dementia. A comparison with radioisotope encephalography. *European Neurology*, 1971, *5*(5), 294–302.

Branconnier, R. J., & Cole, J. O. The impairment index as a symptom-independent parameter of drug efficacy in geriatric psychopharmacology. *Journal of Gerontology*, 1978, *33*(2), 217–223.

Carmichael, J., & Linn, M. W. Functioning of the elderly patient in relation to the physician's diagnosis of chronic brain syndrome. *Journal of the American Geriatrics Society,* 1974, *22*(5), 217–221.

Claessens, W. L., & Wijnen, J. T. The value of vitamin B12 determinations as a routine study method. *Nederlands Tijdschrift voor Geneeskunde,* 1977, *121*(49), 1949–1952.

Cole, M., Kraehenbuhl, B., & Richard, J. Differentiation of the dementias of old age by ultrasonic doppler flowmetry: A pilot study. *Journal of the American Geriatrics Society,* 1977, *25*(7), 314–317.

Cooper, J. E., *et al.* Psychiatric diagnosis in New York and London: A comparative study of mental hospital admissions. *Maudsley Monograph No. 20.* 1972.

Copeland, J. R., Kelleher, M. J., Kellett, J. M., Gourlay, A. J., Gurland, B. J., Fleiss, J. L., & Sharpe, L. A semi-structured clinical interview for the assessment of diagnosis and mental state in the elderly: The Geriatric Mental State Schedule. I. Development and reliability. *Psychological Medicine,* 1976, *6*(3), 439–449.

Cowan, D. W., *et al.* A comparative psychometric assessment of psychogeriatric and geriatric patients. *British Journal of Psychiatry,* 1975, *127*, 33–41.

Crookes, T. G. Indices of early dementia on WAIS. *Psychological Reports,* 1974, *34*(3), 734. (Part 1)

Crookes, T. G., & McDonald, K. G. Benton's visual retention test in the differentiation of depression and early dementia. *British Journal of Social and Clinical Psychology,* 1972, *11*, 66–69.

Davies, A. D. M. Measures of mental deterioration in aging and brain damage. In S. S. Chown & L. A. Davison (Eds.), *Interdisciplinary Topics in Gerontology* (Vol. 1), Basel: Karger, 1968.

Davies, G. V. M. The differential diagnosis of the mental disorders of late life. *Medical Journal of Australia,* 1969, *1*, 242–245.

Duckworth, G. S., & Ross, H. Diagnostic differences in psychogeriatric patients in Toronto, New York and London, England. *Canadian Medical Association,* 1975, *112*(7), 847–851.

Eraut, D. Idiopathic hypoparathyroidism presenting as dementia. *British Medical Journal,* 1974, *1*(905), 429–430.

Erickson, R. C., & Scott, M. L. Clinical memory testing: A review. *Psychological Bulletin,* 1977, *6,* 1130–1149.

Faden, A. I., & Townsend, J. J. Myoclonus in Alzheimer disease. A confusing sign. *Archives of Neurology,* 1976, *33*(4), 278–280.

Fauman, M. A. A diagnostic system for organic brain disorders: Critique and suggestion. *Psychiatric Quarterly,* 1977, *49*(3), 173–186.

Fauman, M. A., & Fauman, B. J. The differential diagnosis of organic based psychiatric disturbance in the emergency department. *J.A.C.E.P.,* 1977, *6*(7), 315–323.

Ferris, S., Crook, T., Sathananthan, G., & Gershon, S. Reaction time as a diagnostic measure in senility. *Journal of the American Geriatrics Society,* 1976, *24*(12), 529–533.

Fink, M., Green, M. A., & Bender, M. B. The face-hand test as a diagnostic sign of organic mental syndrome. *Neurology,* 1952, *2,* 48–56.

Fishback, D. B. Mental Status Questionnaire for organic brain syndrome, with a new visual counting test. *Journal of the American Geriatrics Society,* 1977, *25*(4), 167–170.

Fleiss, J., Gurland, B., & Roche, P. D. Distinctions between organic brain syndrome and functional psychiatric disorders: Based on the Geriatric Mental State interview. *International Journal of Aging and Human Development,* 1976, *7*(4), 323–330.

Foley, J. M. Differential diagnosis of the organic mental disorders in elderly patients. *Advances in Behavioral Biology,* 1972, *3,* 153–161.

Folstein, M. F., Folstein, S. E., & McHugh, P. R. "Mini-mental state": A practical method for grading the cognitive state of patients for the clinician. *Journal of Psychiatric Research,* 1975, *12,* 189–198.

Foster, E. M., Kay, D. W., & Bergmann, K. The characteristics of old people receiving and needing domiciliary services: The relevance of psychiatric diagnosis. *Age and Ageing,* 1976, *5*(4), 245–255.

Fox, J. H., & Huckman, M. S. Computerized tomography: A recent advance in evaluating senile dementia. *Geriatrics,* 1975, *30*(11), 97–100.

Fox, J. H., Topel, J. L., & Huckman, M. S. Use of computerized tomography in senile dementia. *Journal of Neurology, Neurosurgery, and Psychiatry,* 1975, *38*(10), 948–953.

Freemon, F. R. Evaluation and treatment of patients with dementia. *Journal of the National Medical Association,* 1977, *69*(5), 307–310.

Gado, M. H., Coleman, R. E., Lee, K. S., Mikhael, M. A., Alderson, P. O., & Archer, C. R. Correlations between computerized transaxial tomography and radionuclide cisternography in dementia. *Neurology,* 1976, *26*(6), 555–560. (Part 1)

Gaitz, C. M., & Baer, P. E. Diagnostic assessment of the elderly: A multifunctional model. *Gerontologist,* 1970, *10,* 47–52.

Georges, D., Lallemand, A., Coustenoble, J., & Loria, Y. Validation by factor analysis of clinical evaluation scale of disorders of cerebral senescence: Use in a therapeutic trial. *Therapie,* 1977, *32*(2), 173–180.

Geraghty, E. G., Sheridan, M. A., & Healy, J. J. Detection of mental disability in the elderly. *Irish Medical Journal,* 1977, *70*(18), 540–542.

Gerhard, L. Morphological findings in the differential diagnosis of cerebral sclerosis and senile dementia. *Verhandlungen der Deutschen Gesellschaft fuer Pathologie,* 1968, *52,* 164–179.

Goldstein, B. J., & Jacobson, S. Clinical evaluation of SKF-14336 in the treatment of psychosis associated with organic brain syndrome. *Diseases of the Nervous System,* 1969, *30,* 37–41.

Goto, Y. Clinical diagnosis of senile dementia: Introduction of diagnostic methods. *Japanese Journal of the Nursing Art,* 1976, *22*(7), 18–24.

Gun, A. Mental impairment in the elderly: Medical-legal assessment. *Journal of the American Geriatrics Society,* 1977, *25*(5), 193–198.

Gurland, B. Assessment of the Mental Health Status of Older Adults. In J. E. Birren & R. B. Sloane (Eds.), *Handbook of Mental Health and Aging.* Englewood Cliffs: Prentice-Hall, in press.

Gurland, B. J. A broad clinical assessment of psychopathology in the aged. In C. Eisdorfer & M. P. Lawton (Eds.), *The Psychology of Adult Development and Aging,* Washington, D.C.: American Psychological Association, 1973.

Gurland, B., Copeland, J., Sharpe, L., & Kelleher, M. The geriatric mental status interview. *International Journal of Aging and Human Development,* 1976, *7*(4), 303–311.

Gurland, B., Fleiss, J., Goldberg, K., Sharpe, L., Copeland, J., Kelleher, M., & Kellett, J. A semi-structured clinical interview for the assessment of diagnosis and mental state in the elderly: The geriatric mental state schedule. II. A factor analysis. *Psychological Medicine,* 1976, *6*(3), 451–459.

Haase, G. R. Diseases presenting as dementia *Contemporary Neurology Series,* 1977, *15,* 27–67.

Hafken, L., Leichter, S., & Reich, T. Organic brain dysfunction as a possible consequence of postgastrectomy hypoglycemia. *American Journal of Psychiatry,* 1975, *132*(12), 1321–1324.

Haglund, R. M. & Schuckit, M. A. A clinical comparison of tests of organicity in elderly patients. *Journal of Gerontology,* 1976, *31*(6), 654–659.

Harenko, A. Electroencephalography in neuro-psychiatric diagnostics of geriatric patients. *Gerontologist,* 1974, *20,* 32-39.

Hartmann, A., & Alberti, E. Differentiation of communicating hydrocephalus and presenile dementia by continuous recording of cerebrospinal fluid pressure. *Journal of Neurology, Neurosurgery, and Psychiatry,* 1977, *40*(7), 630-640.

Howard, A. R. Diagnostic value of the Wechsler Memory Scale with selected groups of institutionalized patients. *Journal of Consulting Psychology,* 1950, *14,* 376-380.

Huckman, M. S., Fox, J. H., & Ramsey, R. G. Computed tomography in the diagnosis of degenerative diseases of the brain. *Seminars in Roentgenology,* 1977, *12,* 63-75.

Huckman, M., Fox, J., & Topel, J. The validity of criteria for the evaluation of cerebral atrophy by computed tomography. *Radiology,* 1975, *116,* 85-92.

Huffer, V. Organic versus functional psychosis: Differential diagnosis. *Maryland State Medical Journal,* 1970, *19*(10), 65-68.

Hughes, C. P., Myers, F. K., Smith, K., & Torack, R. M. Nosologic problems in dementia. A clinical and pathologic study of 11 cases. *Neurology*(Minneapolis), 1973, *23*(4), 344-351.

Hunt, W. L. The relative rate of decline of Wechsler-Bellevue "hold" and "don't hold" tests. *Journal of Consulting Psychology,* 1949, *13,* 440-443.

Irving, G., Robinson, R. A., & McAdam, W. The validity of some cognitive tests in the diagnosis of dementia. *British Journal of Psychiatry,* 1970, *117,* 149-156.

Isaacs, B., & Kennie, A. T. The set test as an aid to the detecttion of dementia in old people. *British Journal of Psychiatry,* 1973, *123*(575), 467-470.

Jacobs, J. W., Bernhard, M. R., Delgado, A., & Strain, J. J. Screening for organic mental syndromes in the medically ill. *Annals of Internal Medicine,* 1977, *86,* 40-46.

Jenkyn, L., Walsh, D., Culver, C., & Reeves, A. Clinical signs in diffuse cerebral dysfunction. *Journal of Neurology, Neurosurgery, and Psychiatry,* 1977, *40*(10), 956–966.

Jonsson, C. O., Waldton, S., & Malhammar, G. The psychiatric symptomatology in senile dementia assessed by means of an interview. *Acta Psychiatrica Scandinavica,* 1972, *48*(2), 103–121.

Kahn, R., Goldfarb, A., Pollack, M., & Peck, A. Brief objective measures for the determination of mental status in the aged. *American Journal of Psychiatry,* 1960, *117,* 326–328.

Kahn, R., Goldfarb, A., Pollack, M., & Gerber, I. The relationship of mental and physical status in institutionalized aged persons. *American Journal of Psychiatry,* 1960, *117*(2), 120–124.

Katzman, R., & Karasu, T. B. Differential diagnosis of dementia. In W. S. Fields, (Ed.), *Neurological and Sensory Disorders in the Elderly.* New York: Stratton, 1975.

Kelleher, M., Copeland, J., Gurland, B., & Sharpe, L. Assessment of the older psychiatric inpatient. *International Journal of Aging and Human Development,* 1976, *7*(4), 295–302.

Kendall, R. E., *et al.* Diagnostic criteria of American and British psychiatrists. *Archives of General Psychiatry,* 1972, *25,* 123–130.

Kiloh, L. G. Pseudo-dementia. *Acta Psychiatrica Scandinavica,* 1961, *37,* 336–351.

Kitzig, M., & Kitzig, P. Examples of syndromes erroneously ascribed to endogenous psychiatric causes eventually revealed as organic brain disease. *Oeff. Gesundheitswes,* 1977, *39*(11), 676–679.

Kleban, M. H., Brody, E. M., & Lawton, M. P. Personality traits in the mentally-impaired aged and their relationship to improvements in current functioning. *Gerontologist,* 1971, *11*(2), 134–140.

Klingner, A., *et al.* A psychogeriatric assessment program: III. Clinical and experimental psychologic aspects. *Journal of the American Geriatrics Society,* 1976, *24,* 17–24.

Kraus, J. A combined test used for the diagnosis of organic brain condition: Predictive validity based on radiographic and electroencephalographic criteria. *Journal of Abnormal Psychology,* 1970, *75*(2), 187–188.

Kuriansky, J., Gurland, B., & Cowan, D. The usefulness of a psychological test battery. *International Journal of Aging and Human Development,* 1976, *7*(4), 331–342.

Lehmann, H. E., & Ban, T. A. Psychometric tests in evaluation of brain pathology response to drugs. *Geriatrics,* 1970, *25*(4), 142–147.

Lowe, G. R. The phenomenology of hallucinations as an aid to differential diagnosis. *British Journal of Psychiatry,* 1973, *123*(577), 621–633.

Lying-Tunell, U., & Marions, O. A triad of airencephalographic findings in patients with mental impairment: A controlled prospective study. *Neuroradiology,* 1975, *9*(5), 251–265.

Martin, W. A. & Smith, A. O. The evaluation of dementia. *Diseases of the Nervous System,* 1974, *35*(6), 262–265.

McConnachie, R. W. The clinical assessment of brain failure in the elderly. *Pharmacology,* 1978, *1,* 27–35. (Supplement 16)

Measures of dementia and senile change. *Lancet,* 1969, *1*(585), 88–89.

Meer, B., & Baker, J. A. The Stockton geriatric rating scale. *Journal of Gerontology,* 1966, *21*(3), 392–403.

Menzer, L., Sabin, T., & Mark, V. H. Computerized axial tomography. Use in the diagnosis of dementia. *Journal of the American Medical Association,* 1975, *234*(7), 754–757.

Muller, H. F., Dastoor, D. P., Hontela, S., Kachanoff, R., & Klingner, A. A psychogeriatric assessment program. IV. Interdisciplinary aspects. *Journal of the American Geriatrics Society,* 1976, *24*(2), 54–57.

Mutsers, A. Differential diagnosis of the psycho-organic syndrome. *Revue Medicale de Liege*(Fre.), 1976, *31*(23), 720–722.

Nathan, P. E., Simpson, H. F., & Andberg, M. M. A systems analytic model of diagnosis. II. The diagnostic validity of abnormal perceptual behavior. *Journal of Clinical Psychology,* 1969, *25*(2), 115–119.

Nathan, P. E., Simpson, H. F., Andberg, M. M., & Patch, V. D. A systems analytic model of diagnosis. III. The diagnostic validity of abnormal cognitive behavior. *Journal of Clinical Psychology,* 1969, *25*(2), 120–130.

Norton, J. C., Romano, P. O., & Sandifer, M. G. The ward function inventory (WFI): A scale for use with geriatric and demented inpatients. *Diseases of the Nervous System,* 1977, *38,* 20–23.

Nott, P. N., & Fleminger, J. J. Presenile dementia: The difficulties of early diagnosis. *Acta Psychiatrica Scandinavica,* 1975, *51*(3), 210–217.

O'Brien, M. D. Some neurological aspects of dementia. *Gerontologia Clinica,* 1971, *13*(6), 339–349.

Overall, J. E., & Gorham, D. R. Organicity versus old age in objective and projective test performance. *Journal of Consulting and Clinical Psychology,* 1972, *39,* 98–105.

Pattie, A. H., & Gilleard, C. J. A brief psychogeriatric assessment schedule: Validation against psychiatric diagnosis and discharge from hospital. *British Journal of Psychiatry,* 1975, *27,* 489–493.

Paulson, G. W. The neurological examination in dementia. *Contemporary Neurology Series,* 1977, *15,* 169–188.

Perez, F. I., Stump, D. A., Gay, J. R., & Hart, V. R. Intellectual performance in multi-infarct dementia and Alzheimer's disease: A replication study. *Canadian Journal of Neurological Science,* 1976, *3*(3), 181–187.

Pfeiffer, E. A short portable mental status questionnaire for the assessment of organic brain deficit in elderly patients. *Journal of the American Geriatrics Society,* 1975, *23*(10), 433–441.

Priest, R. G., Tarighati, S., & Shariatmadari, M. E. A brief test of organic brain disease validation in a mental hospital population. *Acta Psychiatrica Scandinavica,* 1969, *45*(4), 347–354.

Qureshi, K. N., & Hodkinson, H. M. Evaluation of a ten-question mental test in the institutionalized elderly. *Age and Ageing,* 1974, *3*(3), 152–157.

Reid, A. H., & Aungle, P. G. Dementia in aging mental defectives: A clinical psychiatric study. *Journal of Mental Deficiency Research,* 1974, *18,* 15–23.

Reid, R. W., & Youngs, D. D. Second thoughts on dementia. Evaluation and management of patients with mild dementia. *Primary Care,* 1975, *2,* 9–18.

Rosen, H. & Swigar, M. F. Depression and normal pressure hydrocephalus. *Journal of Nervous and Mental Disease,* 1976, *163,* 35–40.

Roth, M. Classification and aetiology in mental disorders of old age: Some recent developments. In D. W. K. Kay & A. Walk (Eds.), *Recent Developments in Psychogeriatrics.* Ashford, Kent, England: Headley, 1971.

Roth, M., & Morrissey, J. D. Problems in the diagnosis and classifications of mental disorders in old age. *Journal of Mental Science,* 1952, *98,* 66–80.

Roth, M., & Myers, D. H. The diagnosis of dementia. In T. Silverstone and B. Barraclough (Eds.), *Contemporary Psychiatry.* Ashford: Headley Brothers, 1976.

Roth, M., & Myers, D. H. The diagnosis of dementia. *British Journal of Psychiatry,* 1975, Spec. No. 9, 87–99.

San Luis, R. R. Simple tests can indicate type of brain damage. *Geriatrics,* 1977, *32*(6), 115–116.

Sata, L. S. Diagnosing organic psychosis. *Maryland State Medical Journal,* 1970, *19*(10), 61–64.

Schaie, K. W., & Schaie, J. P. Clinical assessment and aging. In J. E. Birren & K. W. Schaie (Eds.), *Handbook of the Psychology of Aging.* New York: Van Nostrand Reinhold, 1977.

Seipel, J. H., Fisher, R., Floam, J. E., & Bohm, M. Rheoencephalographic and other studies of betahistine in humans. III. Improved methods of diagnosis and selection in arteriosclerotic dementia. *Journal of Clinical Pharmacology,* 1977, *17*, 63–75.

Shader, R. I., Harmatz, J. S., & Salzman, C. A new scale for clinical assessment in geriatric populations: Sandoz clinical assessment. *Journal of the American Geriatrics Society,* 1974, *22*(3), 107–113.

Shukla, T. R. Pathological verbalization on inkblots and psychodiagnosis. *Indian Journal of Clinical Psychology,* 1976, *3,* 17–21.

Spitzer, R. L., & Fleiss, J. L. A re-analysis of the reliability of psychiatric diagnosis. *British Journal of Psychiatry,* 1974, *125,* 341–347.

Stengel, E. A study of the symptomatology and differential diagnosis of Alzheimer's and Pick's disease. *Journal of Mental Science,* 1943, *89,* 1–20.

Stonier, P. D. Score changes following repeated administration of mental status questionnaires. *Age and Ageing,* 1974, *3*(2), 91–96.

Suchett-Kaye, A. I., Sarkar, U., Elkan, G., & Waring, M. Physical, mental and social assessment of elderly patients suffering from cerebrovascular accident with special reference to rehabilitation. *Gerontologia Clinica,* 1971, *13,* 192–206.

Swallow, M. The diagnosis of dementia. A clinical review. *Irish Journal of Medical Science,* 1973, *142*(3), 132–140.

Thiery, E., Verwerft, E., & Vander Eecken, H. The elizur test of psycho-organicity (adults): A cross-validation study. *Acta Neurologica Belgica,* 1975, *75*(2), 93–98.

Todorov, A. B., Go, R. C., Constantinidis, J., & Elston, R. C. Specificity of the clinical diagnosis of dementia. *Journal of Neurological Sciences,* 1975, *26,* 81–98.

Uncovering physical illness in elderly patients with dementia. *British Medical Journal,* 1977, *2*(6101), 1499–1500.

Ward, N., Rowlett, D., & Burke, P. Sodium amylobarbitone in the differential diagnosis of confusion. *American Journal of Psychiatry,* 1977, *135,* 75–78.

Watson, C. G., Thomas, R. W., Felling, J., & Anderson, D. Differentiation of organics from schizophrenics with the trail making, critical flicker fusion and light intensity matching tests. *Journal of Clinical Psychology,* 1969, *25,* 130–133.

Watson, R. T., & Heilman, K. M. The differential diagnosis of dementia. *Geriatrics,* 1974, *29*(4), 145–147. (Passim)

Weinstein, E. A., Kahn, R. L., Sugarman, L. A., & Linn, L. Diagnostic use of amobarbital sodium (amytal sodium) in organic brain disease. *American Journal of Psychiatry,* 1953, *109,* 889–894.

Wells, C. E. & Buchanan, D. C. The clinical use of psychological testing in evaluation for dementia. *Contemporary Neurology Series,* 1977, *15,* 189–204.

Wells, C. E., & Duncan, G. W. Danger of overreliance on computerized cranial tomography. *American Journal of Psychiatry,* 1977, *134*(7), 811–813.

When is dementia presenile? *British Medical Journal,* 1972, *2*(811), 465.

Wilbert, D. E., Jorstad, V., Loren, J. D., & Wirrer, B. Determination of grave disability. *Journal of Nervous and Mental Disease,* 1976, *162,* 35–39.

Williams, S. E., Bell, D. S., & Gye, R. S. Neurosurgical disease encountered in a psychiatric service. *Journal of Neurology, Neurosurgery and Psychiatry,* 1974, *37*(1), 112–116.

Wyper, D. J., McAlpine, C. J., Jawad, K., & Jennett, B. Effects of a carbonic anhydrase inhibitor on cerebral blood flow on geriatric patients. *Journal of Neurology, Neurosurgery and Psychiatry,* 1976, *39*(9), 885–889.

VI. REHABILITATION AND MANAGEMENT

A. DRUG STUDIES

Abuzzahab, F., Sr., Merwin, G., Zimmermann, R., & Sherman, M. A double-blind investigation of piracetam (nootropil) versus placebo in the memory of geriatric inpatients. *Psychopharmacology Bulletin,* 1978, *14,* 23–25.

Altman, H., Mehta, D., Evenson, R. C., & Sletten, I. W. Behavioral effects of drug therapy on psychogeriatric inpatients. I. Chlorpromazine and thioridazine. *Journal of the American Geriatrics Society,* 1973, *21*(6), 241–248.

Ananth, J. V., Deutsch, M., & Ban, T. A. Senilex in the treatment of geriatric patients. *Current Therapeutic Research,* 1971, *13*(5), 316–321.

Ananth, J. V., Saxena, B. M., Lehmann, H. E., & Ban, T. A. Combined administration of thioridazine and nicotinic acid in the treatment of geriatric patients. *Current Therapeutic Research,* 1971, *13*(3), 158–161.

Bambasova, E., Bilkova, J., & Budinska, K. Papaverin in the treatment of geriatric patients. *Act. Nerv. Super.*(Praha), 1974, *16*(3), 191–192.

Ban, T. A. Geriatric psychopharmacology: Clinical evaluation of brain function in the aged. *Psychopharmacology Bulletin,* 1978, *14,* 20–22.

Ban, T. A. Psychopathology, psychopharmacology and the organic brain syndromes. Part I. *Psychosomatics,* 1976, *17*(2), 77–82.

Ban, T. A., *et al.* Differential effects of trazodone in depressed, schizophrenic and geriatric patients. *International Journal of Clinical Pharmacology,* 1974, *9,* 23–27.

Bazo, A. J. An ergot alkaloid preparation (hydergine) versus papaverine in treating common complaints of the aged: Double-blind study. *Journal of the American Geriatrics Society,* 1973, *21*(2), 63–71.

Birkett, D. P. Vasodilators in geriatric psychiatry. *Journal of the Medical Society of New Jersey,* 1971, *68*(8), 619–623.

Birkett, D. P., & Boltuch, B. Chlorpromazine in geriatric psychiatry. *Journal of the American Geriatrics Society,* 1972, *20*(8), 403–406.

Birkett, D. P., Hirschfield, W., & Simpson, G. M. Thiothixene in the treatment of diseases of the senium. *Current Therapeutic Research,* 1972, *14*(12), 775–779.

Boiullat, J. E., Saxena, B. M., Lehmann, H. E., & Ban, T. A. Combined administration of thioridazine, nicotinic acid, and fluoxymesterone in the treatment of geriatric patients. *Current Therapeutic Research,* 1971, *13*(8), 541–544.

Bower, H. M., & McDonald, C. A controlled trial of A.N.P. 235 (lucidril) in senile dementia. *Medical Journal of Australia,* 1966, *2*(6), 270–271.

Boyd, W. D., Graham-White, J., Blackwood, G., Glen, I., & McQueen, J. Clinical effects of choline in Alzheimer senile dementia (letter). *Lancet,* 1977, *2*(8040), 711.

Branchey, M. H., Lee, J. H., Simpson, G. M., Elgart, B., & Vicencio, A. Loxapine succinate in a neuroleptic agent: Evaluation in two populations of elderly psychiatric patients. *Journal of the American Geriatrics Society,* 1978, *26*(6), 263–267.

Branconnier, R. J., Cole, J. O., & Gardos, G. ACTH4-10 in the amelioration of neuropsychological symptomatology associated with senile organic brain syndrome. *Psychopharmacology Bulletin,* 1978, *14,* 27–30.

Branconnier, R., & Cole, J. O. Senile dementia and drug therapy. In K. Nandy & I. Sherwin (Eds.), *The Aging Brain and Senile Dementia.* New York: Plenum Press, 1977.

Brodie, N. H. A double-blind trial of naftidrofuryl in treating confused elderly patients in general practice. *Practitioner,* 1977, *218*(1304), 274–279.

Broe, G. A., & Caird, F. I. Levodopa for parkinsonism in elderly and demented patients. *Medical Journal of Australia,* 1973, *1*(13), 630–635.

Burian, E. An ergot alkaloid preparation (hydergine) in the treatment of presenile brain atrophy (Alzheimer's disease): Case report. *Journal of the American Geriatrics Society,* 1974, *22*(3), 126–128.

Cahn, L. A., & Diesfeldt, H. F. The use of neuroleptics in the treatment of dementia in old age. A critical analysis with reference to an experiment with a long-acting oral neuroleptic (penfluridol janssen). *Psychiatria, Neurologia, Neurochirurgia,* 1973, *76*(6), 411–420.

Chynoweth, R., & Foley, J. Presenile dementia responding to steroid therapy. *British Journal of Psychiatry,* 1969, *115* (523), 703–708.

Cia Madariaga, F. M., Rud, C., Rovira, B., Mantilaro, E., Alvarez, O., Baretic, E., & Moro, R. Preliminary report on the treatment of dementia syndromes with levodopa. *Prensa Medica Argentina,* 1971, *57*(46), 2098–2102.

Cohen, W. J., & Cohen, N. H. Lithium carbonate, haloperidol, and irreversible brain damage. *Journal of the American Medical Association,* 1974, *230*(9), 1283–1287.

Colafelice, M., Castellani, A., & Perbellini, D. Senile, presenile and arteriosclerotic dementia. Psychological and laboratory aspects studied in the light of treatment with neurohomologous phospholipids. *Acta Neurologia*(Napoli), 1977, *32*(3), 332–339.

Covington, J. S. Alleviating agitation, apprehension, and related symptoms in geriatric patients: A double-blind comparison of a phenothiazine and a benzodiazepine. *Southern Medical Journal,* 1975, *68*(6), 719–724.

Culebras, A. Effect of papaverine on cerebral electrogenesis. *Neurology,* 1976, *26*(7), 673–679.

Czerwinski, A. W., Clark, M. L., Serafetinides, E. A., Perrier, C., & Huber, W. Safety and efficacy of zinc sulfate in geriatric patients. *Clinical Pharmacology and Therapeutics,* 1974, *15*(4), 436–441.

Danto, B. L. Triflupromazine versus pentylenetetrazol-nicotinic acid for treatment of chronic brain disease in a general hospital psychiatric service. *Journal of the American Geriatrics Society,* 1969, *17*(4), 414–420.

Davies, G., Hamilton, S., Hendrickson, E., Levy, R., & Post, F. The effect of cyclandelate in depressed and demented patients: A controlled study in psychogeriatric patients. *Age and Ageing,* 1977, *6*(3), 156–162.

Dawson-Butterworth, K. The chemopsychotherapeutics of geriatric sedation. *Journal of the American Geriatrics Society,* 1970, *18*(2), 97–114.

Deapril-ST for senile dementia. *Med. Lett. Drugs Therapy,* 1977, *19*(15), 61–62.

Deutsch, M., Saxena, B. M., Lehmann, H. E., & Ban, T. A. Combined administration of thioridazine and fluoxymesterone in the treatment of geriatric patients. *Current Therapeutic Research,* 1970, *12*(2), 805–809.

Drugs for dementia. *Drug and Therapeutics Bulletin,* 1975, *13*(22), 85–87.

Drugs for improvement of cerebral function in the elderly. *Med. Lett. Drugs Therapy,* 1976, *18*(9), 38–39.

Easton, H. G. Letter: Cerebral vasodilators. *British Medical Journal,* 1975, *2*(5964), 195.

Etienne, P., *et al.* Clinical effects of choline in Alzheimer's disease (letter). *Lancet,* 1978, *1*(8062), 508–509.

Fann, W. E., Wheless, J. C., & Richman, B. W. Treating the aged with psychotropic drugs. *Gerontologist,* 1976, *16*(4), 322–328.

Ferm, L. Behavioral activities in demented geriatric patients. Study based on evaluations made by nursing staff members and on patients' scores on a simple psychometric test. *Gerontologia Clinica,* 1974, *16*(4), 185–194.

Ferris, S. H., Sathananthan, G., Gershon, S., & Clark, C. Senile dementia: Treatment with deanol. *Journal of the American Geriatrics Society,* 1977, *25*(6), 241–244.

Gaitz, C. M., Varner, R. V., & Overall, J. E. Pharmacotherapy for organic brain syndrome in late life. Evaluation of an ergot derivative vs. placebo. *Archives of General Psychiatry,* 1977, *34*(7), 839–845.

Gedye, J. L., Exton-Smith, A. N., & Wedgwood, J. A method for measuring mental performance in the elderly and its use in a pilot clinical trial of meclofenoxate in organic dementia (preliminary communication). *Age and Ageing,* 1972, *1*(2), 74–80.

Goldstein, S. E. & Birnbom, F. Piperacetazine versus thioridazine in the treatment of organic brain disease: A controlled double-blind study. *Journal of the American Geriatrics Society,* 1976, *24*(8), 355–358.

Gottfries, C. G., & Gottfries, I. Antinuclear factors in the relation to age, sex, mental disease and treatment with phenothiazines. *Acta Psychiatrica Scandinavica,* 1974, *255,* 193–201. (Supplement)

Grad, B., & Kral, V. A. The delayed effect of ACTH administration on the plasma corticoid level of normal elderly persons and patients with chronic brain syndrome. *Journal of the American Geriatrics Society,* 1969, *17,* 15–24.

Gustafson, L., Risberg, J., Johanson, M., Fransson, M., & Maximilian, V. A. Effects of piracetam on regional cerebral blood flow and mental functions in patients with organic dementia. *Psychopharmacology,* 1978, *56*(2), 115–117.

Hall, P. Cyclandelate in the treatment of cerebral arteriosclerosis. *Journal of the American Geriatric Society,* 1976, *24,* 41–44.

Hall, P., & Harcup, M. A trial of lipotropic enzymes in atheromatous (arteriosclerotic) dementia. *Angiology,* 1969, *20*(5), 287–300.

Harenko, A. Comparison between chlormethiazole and nitrazepam as hypnotics in psycho-geriatric patients. *Current Medical Research and Opinion,* 1975, *2*(10), 657–663.

Haskovec, L., Hynek, K., Jirak, R., & Srutova, K. The action of pyrithioxine in patients with organic encephalopathies. *Act Nerv Super*(Praha), 1973), *15*(2), 121–122.

Hoyer, S., Oesterreich, K., & Stoll, K. D. Effect of pyritinol-GCL on blood flow and oxidative metabolism of the brain in patients with dementia. *Arzneimittel-Forschung,* 1977, *27*(3), 671–674.

Hughes, J. T., Williams, J. G., & Currier, R. D. An ergot alkaloid preparation (Hydergine) in the treatment of dementia: Critical review of the clinical literature. *Journal of the American Geriatrics Society,* 1976, *24*(11), 490–497.

Jarvik, M. E., Gritz, E. R., & Schneider, N. G. Drugs and memory disorders in human aging. *Behavioral Biology,* 1972, *7*(5), 643–648.

Judge, T. G. Drugs and dementia. *British Journal of Clinical Pharmacology,* 1976, *3,* 81–82. (Supplement 1)

Judge, T. G., & Urquhart, A. Naftidrofuryl: a double blind cross-over study in the elderly. *Current Medical Research Opinion,* 1972, *1*(3), 166-172.

Kristensen, V., Olsen, M., & Theilgaard, A. Levodopa treatment of presenile dementia. *Acta Psychiatrica Scandinavica,* 1977, *55,* 41-51.

Kumpel, Q., & Mocek, M. The dynamic of psychotropic drug prescriptions in a gerontopsychiatric ward. *Act Nerv Super* (Praha), 1973, *15*(2), 157-158.

Labrecque, D. C., & Goldberg, R. I. A double-blind study of pentylenetetrazol combined with niacin in senile patients. *Current Therapeutic Research,* 1967, 9(12), 611-617.

Leckman, J., Ananth, J. V., Ban, T. A., & Lehmann, H. E. Pentylenetetrazol in the treatment of geriatric patients with disturbed memory function. *Journal of Clinical Pharmacology,* 1971, *11*(4), 301-303.

Lehmann, H. E., & Ban, T. A. CNS stimulants and anabolic substances in geropsychiatric therapy. *Psychopharmacology Bulletin,* 1975, *11*(4), 51.

Lehmann, H. E., Ban, T. A., & Saxena, B. M. Nicotinic acid, thioridazine, fluoxymenterone and their combinations in hospitalized geriatric patients: A systematic clinical study. *Canadian Psychiatric Association,* 1972, *17*(4), 315-320.

Levine, F. M., Spitalnik, R., & Dobos, C. Caudate nucleus effects on geriatric senility: Effect of belladonna on learning and memory of geriatric patients. *Perceptual and Motor Skills,* 1973, *37*(3), 1003-1007.

Lewis, C., Ballinger, B., & Presly, A. Trial of levodopa in senile dementia. *British Medical Journal,* 1978, *1*(6112), 550.

Lloyd-Evans, S., Brocklehurst, J. C., & Palmer, M. K. Assessment of drug therapy in chronic brain failure. *Gerontology,* 1978, *24*(4), 304-311.

March, J., Field, J., Shanley, J., & Turner, W. J. Biochemical observations during a trial of inosiplex in senile dementia. *Journal of the American Geriatrics Society,* 1973, *21*(8), 372-378.

McConnachie, R. W. A clinical trial comparing 'hydergine' with placebo in the treatment of cerebrovascular insufficiency in elderly patients. *Current Medical Research and Opinion,* 1973, *1*(8), 463–468.

McDonald, C., Mowbray, R. M., & Wilson, J. M. A sequential trial of amylobarbitone sodium used as sedation for confused female psychogeriatric patients. *Gerontologia Clinica,* 1970, *12*(6), 335–338.

Meyer, J., Welch, K., Deshmukh, V., Perez, F., Jacob, R., Haufrect, D., Mathew, N., & Morrell, R. Neurotransmitter precursor amino acids in the treatment of multi-infarct dementia and Alzheimer's disease. *Journal of the American Geriatrics Society,* 1977, *25*(7), 289–298.

Munch-Petersen, S., Pakkenberg, H., Kornerup, H., Ortmann, J., Ipsen, E., Jacobsen, P., & Simmelsgard, H. RNA treatment of dementia. A double-blind study. *Acta Neurologica Scandinavica,* 1974, *50*(5), 553–572.

Nair, N. P., Ban, T. A., Hontela, S., & Clarke, R. Trazodone in the treatment of organic brain syndromes, with special reference to psychogeriatrics. *Current Therapeutic Research,* 1973, *15*(10), 769–775.

Parkes, J. D., *et al.* Parkinson's disease, cerebral arteriosclerosis, and senile dementia. Clinical features and response to levodopa. *Quarterly Journal of Medicine,* 1974, *43*(169), 49–61.

Phuapradit, P., Phillips, M., Lees, A. J., & Stern, G. M. Bromocriptine in presenile dementia (letter). *British Medical Journal,* 1978, *1*(6119), 1052–1053.

Predescu, V., *et al.* Hydergine-thioridazine combination in the treatment of psychopathological states in old age. *Act. Nerv. Super.,* 1974, *16*(3), 237–238.

Prien, R. F., & Caffey, E. M., Jr. Pharmacologic treatment of elderly patients with organic brain syndrome: a survey of twelve Veterans Administration hospitals. *Comprehensive Psychiatry,* 1977, *18*(6), 551–560.

Rada, R. T. & Kellner, R. Thiothixene in the treatment of geriatric patients with chronic organic brain syndrome. *Journal of the American Geriatrics Society,* 1976, *24*(3), 105–107.

Rada, R. T., & Kellner, R. The effects of thiothixene in geriatric patients with chronic organic brain syndrome. *Psychopharmacology Bulletin,* 1976, *12*(2), 30–32.

Rao, D., Georgiev, E., Paul, P., & Guzman, A. Cyclandelate in the treatment of senile mental changes: A double-blind evaluation. *Journal of the American Geriatrics Society,* 1977, *25*(12), 548–551.

Ratner, J., Rosenberg, G., Kral, V. A., & Engelsmann, F. Anticoagulant therapy for senile dementia. *Journal of the American Geriatrics Society,* 1972, *20*(11), 556–559.

Reed, M. Psychopharmacology in the geriatric patient. *Rocky Mountain Medical Journal,* 1971, *68*(7), 44–48.

Rehman, S. A. Two trials comparing 'hydergine' with placebo in the treatment of patients suffering from cerebrovascular insufficiency. *Current Medical Research and Opinion,* 1973, *1*(8), 456–462.

Rivera, V. M., Meyer, J. S., Baër, P. E., Faibish, G. M., Mathew, N. T., & Hartmann, A. Vertebrobasilar arterial insufficiency with dementia. Controlled trials of treatment with betahistine hydrochloride. *Journal of the American Geriatrics Society,* 1974, *22*(9), 397–406.

Rosen, H. J. Mental decline in the elderly: Pharmacotheraphy (ergot alkaloids versus papaverine). *Journal of the American Geriatrics Society,* 1975, *23*(4), 169–174.

Russell, B. Letter: Drugs and "dementia" in the elderly. *British Medical Journal,* 1973, *4*(895), 783.

Sacks, O. W., Messeloff, C., Schwartz, W., Goldfarb, A., & Kohl, M. Effects of L-Dopa in patients with dementia. *Lancet,* 1970, *658*, 1231.

Scholing, W. E., & Clausen, H. D. Psychological studies of a long-term treatment of the neurovascular syndrome with trivastal (author's translation). *Medizinische Klinik,* 1975, *70*(38), 1522–1527.

Seipel, J., Fisher, R., Floam, J., & Bohm, M. Rheoencephalographic and other studies of betahistine in humans: II. The cerebral and peripheral microcirculatory effects of single doses in geriatric patients with dementia. *Journal of Clinical Pharmacology,* 1975, *15*(2–3), 155–162.

Serentil for chronic brain syndrome. *Med. Lett. Drugs Therapy,* 1975, *17*(16), 68.

Shimamoto, T., Murase, H., & Numano, F. Treatment of senile dementia and cerebellar disorders with phthalazinol. Cyclic AMP increasing agent, phthalazinol, in therapeutic trials in hitherto incurable morbid conditions(I). *Mechanisms of Ageing and Development,* 1976, *5*(4), 241–250.

Shulman, R. The present status of vitamin B 12 and folic acid deficiency in psychiatric illness. *Canadian Psychiatric Association Journal,* 1972, *17*(3), 205–216.

Silverman, G. Management of the elderly agitated demented patient (letter). *British Medical Journal,* 1977, *2*(6082), 318–319.

Smith, G. R., Taylor, C. W., & Linkous, P. Haloperidol versus thioridazine for the treatment of psychogeriatric patients: A double-blind clinical trial. *Psychosomatics,* 1974, *15*(3), 134–138.

Spillane, J. A., Goodhart, M. J., White, P., Bowen, D. M., & Davison, A. N. Choline in Alzheimer's disease (letter). *Lancet,* 1977, *2*(8042), 826–827.

Steginink, A. J. The clinical use of piracetam, a new nootropic drug. The treatment of symptoms of senile involution. *Arzneimittel-Forschung,* 1972, *22*(6), 975–977.

Szobor, A., & Klein, M. Clinical responses to cinnarizin in various psychiatric syndromes. *Therapia Hungarica,* 1973, *21*, 31–34.

Tammaro, A., Noto, M., Mule, M., & Bonaccorso, O. Senile mental deterioration: therapeutic aspects. *Clin. Ter.*(It.), 1975, *72*, 55–65.

Tewfik, G. I., Jain, V. K., Harcup, M., & Magowan, S. Effectiveness of various tranquilizers in the management of senile restlessness. *Gerontologia Clinica,* 1970, *12*(6), 351–359.

Thibault, A. A double-blind evaluation of 'hydergine' and placebo in the treatment of patients with organic brain syndrome and cerebral arteriosclerosis in a nursing home. *Current Medical Research and Opinion,* 1974, *2*(8), 482–487.

Tobin, J. M., Brousseau, E. R., & Lorenz, A. A. Clinical evaluation of haloperidol in geriatric patients. *Geriatrics,* 1970, *25*(6), 119–122.

Trabant, R., Poljakovic, Z., & Trabant, D. Effect of piracetam on the brain-organic psychosyndrome in cerebrovascular insufficiency. Results of a double-blind study in 40 cases. *Therapie der Gegenwart,* 1977, *116*(8), 1504–1521.

Tsuang, M. M., Lu, L. M., Stotsky, B. A., & Cole, J. O. Haloperidol versus thioridazine for hospitalized psychogeriatric patients: Double-blind study. *Journal of the American Geriatrics Society,* 1971, *19*(7), 593–600.

Turek, I., Kurland, A. A., Ota, K. Y., & Hanlon, T. E. Effects of pipradrol hydrochloride on geriatric patients. *Journal of the American Geriatrics Society,* 1969, *17*(4), 408–413.

Van Woert, M. H., Heninger, G., Rathey, U., & Bowens, M. B., Jr. L-dopa in senile dementia. *Lancet,* 1970, *1*(646), 573–574.

Vann, D. Vitamin B12, folic acid, and the care of mentally disturbed aged patients. *Medical Journal of Australia,* 1972, *2*(20), 1149.

Voltolina, E. J., Thompson, S. I., & Tisue, J. Acute organic brain syndrome with propranolol. *Clinical Toxicology,* 1971, *4*(3), 357–359.

Wahl, P. R. Psychosocial implications of disorientation in the elderly. *Nurs. Clin. of North America,* 1976, *11,* 145–155.

Walsh, A. C. Hypochondriasis associated with organic brain syndrome: A new approach to therapy. *Journal of the American Geriatrics Society,* 1976, *24*(9), 430–431.

Walsh, A. C. Prevention of senile and presenile dementia by bishydroxycoumarin (dicumarol) therapy. *Journal of the American Geriatrics Society,* 1969, *17*(5), 477–487.

Walsh, A. C., & Walsh, B. H. Presenile dementia: Further experience with an anticoagulant-psychotherapy regimen. *Journal of the American Geriatrics Society,* 1974, *22*(10), 467–472.

Walsh, A. C., & Walsh, B. H. Senile and presenile dementia: Further observations on the benefits of a dicumarol-psychotherapy regimen. *Journal of the American Geriatrics Society,* 1972, *20*(3), 127–131.

Webb, W. L., Jr. The use of psychopharmacological drugs in the aged. *Geriatrics,* 1971, *26*(6), 94–103.

Westreich, G., Alter, M., & Lundgren, S. Effect of cyclandelate on dementia. *Stroke,* 1975, *6*(5), 535–538.

Will, J., Abuzzahab, F., Sr., & Zimmermann, R. The effects of ACTH4-10 versus placebo in the memory of symptomatic geriatric volunteers. *Psychopharmacology Bulletin,* 1978, *14,* 25–27.

Wyper, D. J., McAlpine, C. J., Jawad, K., & Jennett, B. Effects of a carbonic anhydrase inhibitor on cerebral blood flow in geriatric patients. *Journal of Neurology, Neurosurgery and Psychiatry,* 1976, *39*(9), 885–889.

Young, L. D., Taylor, I., & Holstrom, V. Lithium treatment of patients with affective illness associated with organic brain symptoms. *American Journal of Psychiatry,* 1977, *134*(12), 1405–1407.

Zwerling, I., Plutchik, R., Hotz, M., Kling, R., Rubin, L., Grossman, J., & Siegel, S. B. Effects of a procaine preparation (Gerovital H3) in hospitalized geriatric patients: A double-blind study. *Journal of the American Geriatrics Society,* 1975, *23*(8), 355–359.

B. BEHAVIORAL AND COMMUNITY STUDIES

Aldrich, C. K., & Mendkoff, E. Relocation of the aged and disabled: A mortality study. *Journal of the American Geriatrics Society,* 1963, *11*, 185–194.

Allen, K. S. A group experience for elderly patients with organic brain syndrome. *Health and Social Work,* 1976, *1*(4), 61–69.

Anderson, F. The prevention of senility. *R. Soc. Health Journal,* 1968, *88*(6), 294–298.

Anderson, J. F. A study of disturbed behaviour in patients with dementia in two hospital populations. *Gerontologia Clinica*(Basel), 1970, *12*, 49–64.

Arie, T. Dementia in the elderly: Management. *British Medical Journal,* 1973, *4*(892), 602–604.

Ben Yishay, Y., & Diller, L. Changing of atmospheric environment to improve mental and behavioral function. Applications in treatment of senescence. *New York State Journal of Medicine,* 1973, *73*(24), 2877–2880.

Ben-Yishay, Y., Diller, L., Reich, T., Rosenblum, J. A., & Rusk, H. A. Can oxygen reverse symptoms of senility? *New York State Journal of Medicine,* 1978, *78*(6), 914–919.

Berger, L. F. Activating a psychogeriatric group. *Psychiatrics,* 1978, *50*, 63–66.

Bergmann, K., Foster, E., Justice, A., & Matthews, V. Management of the demented elderly patient in the community. *British Journal of Psychiatry,* 1978, *132*, 441–449.

Bollinger, R. L. Geriatric speech pathology. *Gerontologist,* 1974, *14*(3), 217–220.

Broaddus, S. L. Rehabilitation goals for the elderly psychotic patient: A case history. *Journal of Geriatric Psychiatry,* 1973, 6(2), 243–250.

Brody, E. M., Kleban, M. H., Lawton, M. P., & Silverman, H. A. Excess disabilities of mentally impaired aged: Impact of individualized treatment. *Gerontologist,* 1971, *11*(2), 124–133.

Brook, P., Degun, G., & Mather, M. Reality orientation, a therapy for psychogeriatric patient: A controlled study. *British Journal of Psychiatry,* 1975, *127,* 42–45.

Burnside, I. M. Caring for the aged: Touching is talking. *American Journal of Nursing,* 1973, *73*(12), 2060–2063.

Burnside, I. M. Reality testing: An important concept. *A.R.N. Journal,* 1977, *2*(3), 1–4.

Care of elderly people with dementia. *British Medical Journal,* 1973, *1*(851), 434.

Citrin, R. S., & Dixon, D. N. Reality orientation. A milieu therapy used in an institution for the aged. *Gerontologist,* 1977, *17,* 39–43.

Davidson, S. M., & Nicholas, M. Day treatment for the elderly mentally infirm (letter). *British Medical Journal,* 1977, *1*(6067), 1030.

Degun, G. Reality orientation. A multi-disciplinary therapeutic approach. *Nursing Times,* 1976, *72*(33), 117–120. (Supplement)

Delwaide, P. J., & Gyselynck-Mambourg, A. M. Therapeutic approach to the psycho-organic syndrome. *Revue Medicale de Liege*(Fre.), 1976, *31*(23), 726–728.

Dennis, H. Remotivation therapy for the elderly: A surprising outcome. *Journal of Gerontological Nursing,* 1976, *2*(6), 28–30.

Di Scipio, W. J., & Greenberg, I. M. A specialized neuropsychiatric service in a state hospital. *Hospital Community Psychiatry,* 1971, *22*(4), 104–108.

Eisdorfer, C., & Stotsky, B. Intervention, treatment and rehabilitation of psychiatric disorders. In J. E. Birren & K. W. Schaie (Eds.), *Handbook of the Psychology of Aging.* New York: Van Nostrand Reinhold, 1977.

Eisner, D. A. Can hyperbaric oxygenation improve cognitive functioning in the organically impaired elderly? A critical review. *Journal of Geriatric Psychiatry,* 1975, *8*(2), 173–188.

Eliseo, T. S. Three examples of hypnosis in the treatment of organic brain syndrome with psychosis. *International Journal of Clinical and Experimental Hypnosis,* 1974, *22,* 9–19.

Elmore, J. L. Psychiatric aspects of care of the aged. *North Carolina Medical Journal,* 1967, *28*(9), 379–382.

Fields, G. J. Senility and remotivation: Hope for the senile? *Journal of Long Term Care Administration,* 1976, *4*(3), 1–9.

Fine, F., & Walker, D. J. Management of the elderly agitated demented patient (letter). *British Medical Journal,* 1977, *2*(6086), 580.

Gaitz, C. M., & Baer, P. E. Placement of elderly psychiatric patients. *Journal of the American Geriatrics Society,* 1971, *19*(7), 601–613.

Gelperin, E. A. Rehabilitative psychiatric nursing for chronically ill, elderly patients. *Journal of the American Geriatrics Society,* 1973, *21*(12), 566–568.

Ginsburg, R., & Weintraub, M. Caffeine in the "sundown syndrome." Report of negative results. *Journal of Gerontology,* 1976, *31*(4), 419–420.

Godber, C. The physician and the confused elderly patient. *Journal of the Royal College of Physicians of London,* 1975, *10,* 101–112.

Goga, J. A., & Hambacher, W. O. Treatment approaches with the psychiatric elderly. *Journal of the American Geriatrics Society,* 1977, *25*(7), 328–330.

Goldfarb, A. I., Hochstadt, N. J., Jacobson, J. H., & Weinstein, E. A. Hyperbaric oxygen treatment of organic mental syndrome in aged persons. *Journal of Gerontology,* 1972, *27*(2), 212–217.

Goldstein, S. Community psychiatry and the elderly. *Canadian Medical Association,* 1973, *108*(5), 579–584.

Gordon, M. Implementing the definition of nursing practice: Case study. II. Nursing intervention for the patient with chronic organic brain disease. *Journal of the New York State Nurses Association,* 1975, 6, 20–26.

Guidelines for hospitalization of the "simple senile." *American Journal of Psychiatry,* 1974, *131*(4), 472–474.

Hamada, S. Socio-psychiatric problems of the aging. A practical approach to the community care of the senile mental disturbances (author's translation). *Psychiatria et Neurologia Japonica,* 1976, *78*(10), 653–660.

Handy, I. A. Treatment of the geriatric patient through the interdisciplinary approach. *American Correctional Therapy Journal,* 1970, *24*(2), 54–58.

Harris, C. S., & Ivory, P. B. An outcome evaluation of reality orientiation therapy with geriatric patients in a state mental hospital. *Gerontologist,* 1976, *16*(6), 496–503.

Harris, S., Snyder, B., Snyder, R., & MaGraw, B. Behavior modification therapy with elderly demented patients: Implementation and ethical considerations. *Journal of Chronic Diseases,* 1977, *30*(3), 129–134.

Hartelius, H. Care of senile dementia patients. *Lakartidningen,* 1978, *75*(21), 2113–2114.

Heilman, K. M., & Wilder, B. J. Evaluation and treatment of chronic simple dementias. *Modern Treatment,* 1971, *8*(2), 219–230.

Hillman, D. Stimulation of the long-stay and psychogeriatric patient. *Nursing Times,* 1976, *72*(42), 1648–1649.

Holden, U. P., & Sinebruchow, A. Reality orientation therapy: A study investigating the value of this therapy in the rehabilitation of elderly people. *Age and Ageing,* 1978, 7(2), 83–90.

Hyperbaric oxygen and senile psychosis. *Lancet,* 1969, 2(634), 1348.

Isler, C. Who says senile geriatric patients are untreatable? *RN,* 1975, *38*(6), 40; 42.

Jacobs, E. A., Alvis, J. J., & Small, S. M. Hyperoxygenation: A central nervous system activator? *Journal of Geriatric Psychiatry,* 1972, 5(2), 107–136.

Jarpe, S. Presenile dementia and hydrocephalus. Therapeutic experiences. *Acta Neurologica Scandinavica,* 1970, 46, (Supplement 43:89).

Jolley, D. Hospital inpatient provision for patients with dementia. *British Medical Journal,* 1977, *1*(6072), 1335–1336.

Katz, M. M. Behavioral change in the chronicity pattern of dementia in the institutional geriatric resident. *Journal of the American Geriatrics Society,* 1976, *24*(11), 522–528.

Kent, E. A. Possible organic factors in the prevention of emotional problems of the aged. *Journal of the American Geriatrics Society,* 1975, *23*(12), 541–544.

Kleban, M. H., Brody, E. M., & Lawton, M. P. Personality traits in the mentally-impaired aged and their relationship to improvements in current functioning. *Gerontologist,* 1971, *11*(2), 134–140.

Kosaka, K. On the therapeutic approach to out-patients with organic dementia based on ageing processes of the brain. *Psychiatria et Neurologia Japonica,* 1976, *78*(10), 719–730.

Krop, H., Block, A., Cohen, E., Croucher, R., & Shuster, J. Neuropsychologic effects of continuous oxygen therapy in the aged. *Chest,* 1977, *72*(6), 737–743.

Lamont, E. S. Dementia: A reappraisal of staff attitudes. *Nursing Times,* 1976, *72*(42), 1646–1648.

Lee, R. E. Reality orientation: Restoring the senile to life. *Journal of Practical Nursing,* 1976, *26*(2), 30–31.

Letcher, P. B., Peterson, L. P., & Scarbrough, D. Reality orientation: A historical study of patient progress. *Hospital and Community Psychiatry,* 1974, *25*(2), 801–803.

Letter: Guidelines for hospitalization of the "simple senile". *American Journal of Psychiatry,* 1974, *131*(4), 472–474.

Management of elderly demented patients (Editorial). *British Medical Journal,* 1977, *1*(6072), 1301.

Manaster, A. Therapy with the "senile" geriatric patient. *International Journal of Group Psychotherapy,* 1972, *22*(2), 250–257.

Mars, G. & Nebuloni, G. Treatment of cerebral vascular insufficiency syndromes in old age. Controlled research by double blind technique. *Giornale di Gerontologia,* 1970, *18*(3), 153–176.

Marsden, C. D., & Harrison, M. J. Outcome of investigation of patients with presenile dementia. *British Medical Journal,* 1972, *2*(808), 249–252.

McNicholas, W. A home for the confused elderly. *Nursing Times,* 1977, *73*(20), 747–749.

Miller, E. The management of dementia: A review of some possibilities. *British Journal of Social and Clinical Psychology,* 1977, *16,* 77–83.

Mishara, B. L., Robertson, B., & Kastenbaum, R. Self-injurious behavior in the elderly. *Gerontologist,* 1973, *13*(3), 311–314.

Munch-Peterson, S. Problems relating to patients with senile dementia. *Acta Psychiatrica Scandinavica,* 1966, *42,* 99. (Supplement 191)

Pearce, J. M. Management of elderly demented patients (letter). *British Medical Journal,* 1977, *1*(6077), 1661–1662.

Philips, D. F. Long-term care: Reality orientation. *Hospitals,* 1973, *47*(13), 46–49. (Passim)

Pollock, D. D., & Liberman, R. P. Behavior therapy of incontinence in demented inpatients. *Gerontologist,* 1974, *14*(6), 488–491.

Powell, R. R. Psychological effects of exercise therapy upon institutionalized geriatric mental patients. *Journal of Gerontology,* 1974, *29*(2), 157–161.

Presdescu, V., *et al.* A multidisciplinary approach to the psychosomatic involution syndrome. *Neurologia Psychiatria* (Bucur), 1976, *14*(2), 85–95.

Preston, T. Caring for the aged: When words fail. *American Journal of Nursing,* 1973, *73*(12), 2064–2066.

Raskin, A., Gershon, S., Crook, T. H., Sathananthan, G., & Ferris, S. The effects of hyperbaric and normobaric oxygen on cognitive impairment in the elderly. *Archives of General Psychiatry,* 1978, *35,* 50–56.

Raskind, M. A., Alvarez, C., Pietrzyk, M., Westerlund, K., & Herlin, S. Helping the elderly psychiatric patient in crisis. *Geriatrics,* 1976, *31*(6), 51–56.

Reichenfeld, H. F., Csapo, K. G., Carriere, L., & Gardner, R. C. Rehabilitative psychiatric nursing for chronically ill, elderly patients. *Journal of the American Geriatrics Society,* 1973, *21*(12), 566–568.

Reichenfeld, J. F., Csapo, K. G., Carriere, L., & Gardner, R. C. Evaluating the effect of activity programs on a geriatric ward. *Gerontologist,* 1973, *13*(3), 305–310.

Reid, R. W., & Youngs, D. D. Second thoughts on dementia. Evaluation and management of patients with mild dementia. *Primary Care,* 1975, *2,* 9–18.

Risdorfer, E. N. Review of results in a geriatric intensive treatment unit: Some prospects. *Journal of the American Geriatrics Society,* 1970, *18,* 47–55.

Roberts, R. E. Nursing care study. Senile dementia and depression, and rehabilitation of the patient. *Nursing Times,* 1975, *71*(49), 1931–1933.

Rosenberg, G. Care of the aged. *Canadian Medical Association Journal,* 1973, *108*(5), 547. (Passim)

Salmon, J. H. Senile and presenile dementia: Ventriculoatrial shunt for symptomatic treatment. *Geriatrics,* 1969, *24*(12), 67–72.

Salzberger, G. J. Long term control of agitation in senile psychosis. *Diseases of the Nervous System,* 1966, *27,* 57–59.

Settle, H. A pilot study in reality orientation for the confused elderly. *Journal of Gerontological Nursing,* 1975, *1*(5), 11–16.

Shenkin, H. A., Greenberg, J., Bouzarth, W. F., Gutterman, P., & Morales, J. O. Ventricular shunting for relief of senile symptoms. *Journal of the American Medical Association,* 1973, *225*(12), 1486–1489.

Sillen, J., Feldshuh, B., Frosch, W., Metchik, E., & Parker, B. A multidisciplinary geriatric unit for the psychiatrically impaired in Bellevue Hospital Center. *Medical Care,* 1974, *12*(9), 766–777.

Snyder, B. D., & Harris, S. Treatable aspects of the dementia syndrome. *Journal of the American Geriatrics Society,* 1976, *24*(4), 179–184.

Stern, F. H. Management of chronic brain syndrome secondary to cerebral arteriosclerosis, with special reference to papaverine hydrochloride. *Journal of the American Geriatrics Society,* 1970, *18*(6), 507–512.

Tanaka, T. Management of senile dementia based on humane interaction: Understanding the problems of the aged. *Japanese Journal of the Nursing Art,* 1976, *22*(7), 32–38.

Taulbee, L. R., & Folsom, J. C. Reality orientation for geriatric patients. *Hospital and Community Psychiatry,* 1966, *17*(5), 133–135.

Thompson, L. W., Davis, G. C., Obrist, W. D., & Heyman, A. Effects of hyperbaric oxygen on behavioral and physiological measures in elderly demented patients. *Journal of Gerontology,* 1976, *31, 23–28.*

Thornton, W. E., & Pray, B. J. Clinical psychiatric approach to dementia. *Journal of the Florida Medical Association,* 1974, *61*(10), 769–770.

Wells, D. A., & Liebowitz, S. W. Psychiatric hospitalization for senile dementia. *Journal of the American Geriatrics Society,* 1972, *20*(8), 391–393.

Wershow, H. J. Comment: Reality orientation for gerontologists. Some thoughts about senility. *Gerontologist,* 1977, *17*(4), 297–302.

Whitehead, J. A. Services for old people with mental symptoms. *Community Health*(Bristol), 1972, 4(2), 83–86.

Yalom, I. D., & Terrazas, F. Group therapy for psychotic elderly patients. *American Journal of Nursing,* 1968, *68*(8), 1690–1694.

Yoshizawa, I. The problem of the treatment for the aged mentally ill from social casework point of view: Centering around the old person in his own home. *Psychiatria et Neurologia Japonica,* 1976, *78*(10), 661–668.

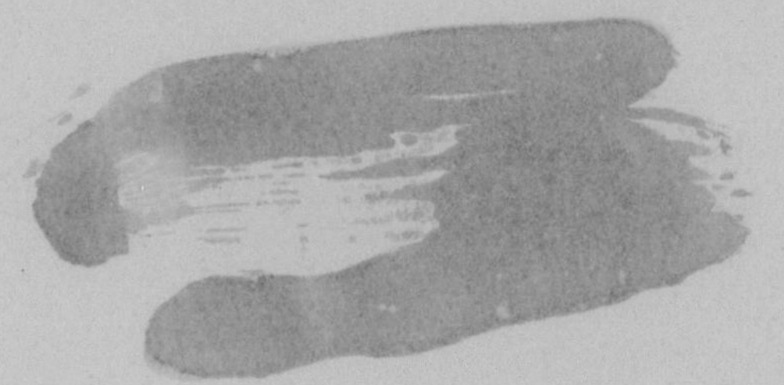